Tips and Tricks for Problem Fractures, Volume I

W0050679

Daniel S. Horwitz • Michael Suk
Teresa K. Swenson
Editors

Tips and Tricks for Problem Fractures, Volume I

The Upper Extremity

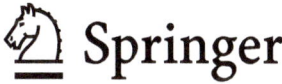

Editors
Daniel S. Horwitz
Department of Orthopaedic
Surgery
Geisinger Health System
Geisinger Musculoskeletal
Institute
Danville, PA
USA

Michael Suk
Department of Orthopedic
Surgery
Geisinger Medical Center
Danville, PA
USA

Teresa K. Swenson
Department of Orthopedic
Surgery
Geisinger Medical Center
Danville, PA
USA

ISBN 978-3-030-38273-5   ISBN 978-3-030-38274-2   (eBook)
https://doi.org/10.1007/978-3-030-38274-2

This Springer imprint is published by the registered company Springer Nature Switzerland AG
The registered company address is: Gewerbestrasse 11, 6330 Cham, Switzerland

Preface

Orthopedic trauma continues to evolve at a rapid pace, based not only on changing technology but also on an expanded knowledge base and an understanding of the healing process. The vast increase in implant options has led to the necessity for continuous learning so that the technical aspects of any given procedure are understood.

In conjunction with this, many instructional courses, both regionally and nationally, have shifted from an emphasis on historical literature and broad topic review to a focus on technical tips and tricks, with the goal of demonstrating how one actually performs a surgical procedure.

This change has been widely praised and, as a result, has led to the development of this text. The goal of *Tips and Tricks for Problem Fractures* is to clearly communicate and visually demonstrate the detailed thought process and required surgical steps in order to avoid complications and achieve excellence, based on the experience of experts in each anatomic area.

While not intended to be comprehensive in any sense, our hope is that experienced surgeons as well as residents in training can review these topics and come away with several "pearls of knowledge" that will aid them in their planning and execution of surgical treatments.

Danville, PA, USA   Daniel S. Horwitz

Contents

Abbreviations

A

AC	Acromioclavicular
AP	Anteroposterior
ATLS	Advanced trauma life support
3D	Three-dimensional

C

CC	Coracoclavicular
CRPP	Closed reduction and percutaneous pinning
CT	Computed tomography

D

DC	Dynamic compression
DIC	Distal intercarpal ligament
DIP	Distal interphalangeal
DISSI	Dorsal intercalated segment instability
DRC	Dorsal radiocarpal
DSSI	Double shoulder suspensory instability

E

ER   Emergency department

F

FCR   Flexor carpi radialis

G

GPA   Glenopolar angle

I

IM   Intramedullary

K

K   Kirschner

L

LC-DCP   Low contact dynamic compression plates
LMA   Laryngeal mask airway
LUCL   Lateral ulnar collateral ligament

M

MCL   Medial collateral ligament
MIPO   Minimally invasive plate osteosynthesis
MRI   Magnetic resonance imaging

O

ORIF   Open reduction internal fixation

P

PIP   Proximal interphalangeal
PRUJ   Proximal radioulnar joint
PT   Physical therapy

R

ROM   Range of motion
RSA   Reverse shoulder arthroplasty

S

SC   Sternoclavicular/scaphocapitate
SL   Scapholunate

T

THC   Triquetrum-hamate-capitate

Contributors

Anil Akoon, MD, MBA Department of Orthopaedic Surgery, Geisinger Health System, Danville, PA, USA

Yelena Bogdan, MD Department of Orthopaedic Surgery, Geisinger – Holy Spirit, Camp Hill, PA, USA

Mark Dunleavy, MD Penn State Health Milton S. Hershey Medical Center, Hershey, PA, USA

C. Liam Dwyer, MD Department of Orthopaedics, Geisinger Medical Center, Danville, PA, USA

Brittany Garcia, MD Department of Orthopaedic Surgery, University of Utah, Salt Lake City, UT, USA

Steven H. Goldberg, MD Department of Orthopaedic Surgery, Geisinger Health System, Danville, PA, USA

Daniel S. Horwitz, MD Department of Orthopaedic Surgery, Geisinger Health System, Geisinger Musculoskeletal Institute, Danville, PA, USA

Jaclyn M. Jankowski, DO Department of Orthopaedic Surgery, Jersey City Medical Center – RWJ Barnabas Health, Jersey City, NJ, USA

Joel Christian Klena, MD Division of Hand Surgery, Department of Orthopaedic Surgery, Geisinger Medical Center, Danville, PA, USA

Frank A. Liporace, MD Division of Orthopaedic Trauma and Adult Reconstruction, Department of Orthopaedic Surgery, Jersey City Medical Center – RWJ Barnabas Health, Jersey City, NJ, USA

Hemil Maniar, MD Musculoskeletal Institute, Geisinger Health System, Danville, PA, USA

Mai P. Nguyen, MD Department of Orthopaedic Surgery, University of Minnesota, Minneapolis, MN, USA

Rodrigo Pesantez, MD Department of Orthopedic Surgery, Fundación Santa Fe de Bogotá, Bogotá, Cundinamarca, Colombia

Damian M. Rispoli, MD Musculoskeletal Institute, Geisinger Health System, Lemoyne, PA, USA

Torre Ruth, MD Department of Orthopaedic Surgery, Geisinger – Holy Spirit, Camp Hill, PA, USA

Daniela Sanchez, MD Musculoskeletal Institute, Geisinger Health System, Danville, PA, USA

Kirsten A. Sumner, MD Department of Orthopaedic Surgery, Geisinger Medical Center, Danville, PA, USA

Heather A. Vallier, MD Department of Orthopaedic Surgery, Case Western Reserve University, Metro Health System, Cleveland, OH, USA

Benjamin Richards Wagner, MD Department of Orthopaedics, Geisinger Medical Center, Danville, PA, USA

Angela A. Wang, MD Department of Orthopaedic Surgery, University of Utah, Salt Lake City, UT, USA

Michael Karl-Heinz Wich, MD Department of Trauma and Orthopedic Surgery, Unfallkrankenhaus Berlin, Berlin, Germany

Richard S. Yoon, MD Division of Orthopaedic Trauma and Adult Reconstruction, Department of Orthopaedic Surgery, Jersey City Medical Center – RWJ Barnabas Health, Jersey City, NJ, USA

Chapter 1
Clavicle Fracture: Open Reduction Internal Fixation

Yelena Bogdan and Torre Ruth

Introduction

Clavicle fractures, particularly those of the midshaft, have traditionally been treated conservatively. However, several studies show improved functional outcomes with early fixation of these fractures though they are tempered by frequent need for plate removal. This section addresses both standard open and minimally invasive approaches to plating of midshaft clavicle fractures, implant choices, and plate placement.

Equipment

Any standard system is amenable to clavicle plating, including various specialty plates and reconstruction plates that can be bent by the surgeon to fit the clavicle. A small

Y. Bogdan (✉) · T. Ruth
Department of Orthopaedic Surgery, Geisinger – Holy Spirit,
Camp Hill, PA, USA
e-mail: ybogdan@geisinger.edu

© Springer Nature Switzerland AG 2020   1
D. S. Horwitz et al. (eds.), *Tips and Tricks for Problem Fractures, Volume I*,
https://doi.org/10.1007/978-3-030-38274-2_1

or mini-fragment set is usually sufficient. For provisional fixation, 1.6 mm Kirschner wires and small reduction forceps can be used. For severely shortened fractures that are not immediately fixed, a mini-distractor can help bring the fracture out to length. If using a reconstruction plate, plate benders (either manual or tabletop) are helpful to contour to the S-shaped clavicle. Bone graft in the form of cancellous chips or other forms according to the surgeon's preference can be available as needed though for most acute fractures it is rarely used.

Positioning

Either the beach chair or a variant of the supine position can be used for clavicle fixation. In both cases, it is preferable to keep the entire arm prepped and available for range of motion throughout the surgery (Fig. 1.1). An arm holder for the beach chair may help bring the distal fragment superiorly, assisting with reduction. In the supine position, a vascular-type table with a central support rather than end support should be used as this will allow the C-arm to be brought in for the appropriate views (inlet and outlet views of the clavicle) at the head of the table (Fig. 1.2).

For the pictured supine position, the table should be placed in slight reverse Trendelenburg for ease of access to the clavicle. A bump can be placed between the scapulae to help bring the clavicle forward [1]. A sloppy lateral position assisted with a beanbag or blankets is also helpful for bringing the operative site closer to the surgeon. The head of the patient should be turned away to the contralateral side in order to allow prepping and draping toward the ipsilateral ear. The medial one-third of the clavicle should be exposed by the drapes, including the sternal notch (Fig. 1.3). Prior to draping, preliminary X-rays should be performed to ensure adequate visualization. The contralateral clavicle should also be accessible for imaging if it is used as a template for plate bending.

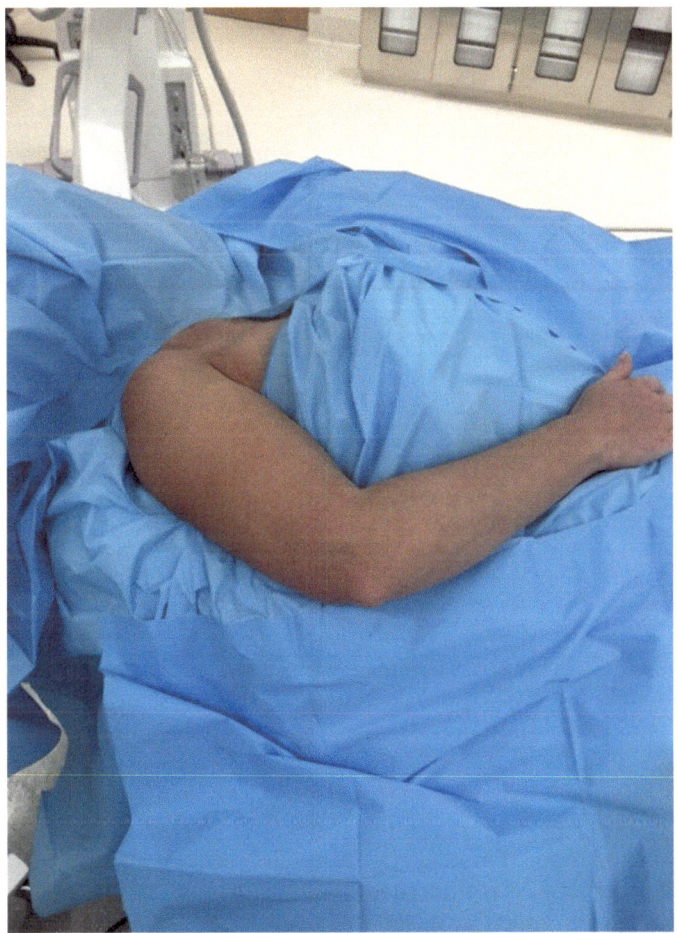

FIGURE 1.1 Supine positioning for clavicle plating. Entire operative arm must be exposed

Approach

The two approaches most frequently used in the literature are the standard open approach and MIPO (minimally invasive plate osteosynthesis). Studies show similar union times in

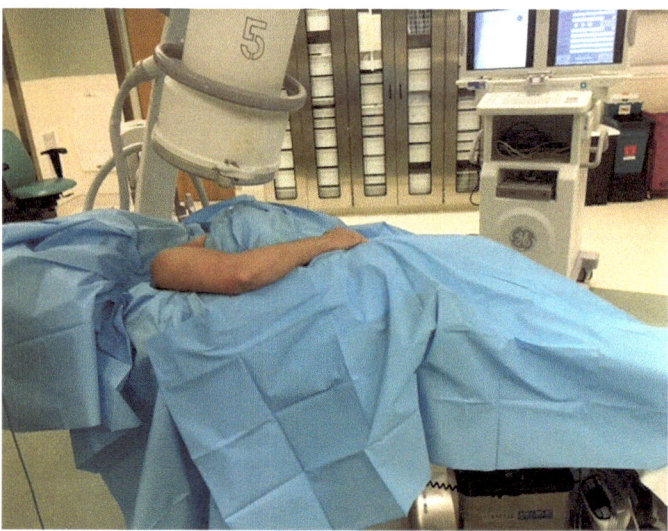

FIGURE 1.2 Use of a table that allows C-arm placement at the head for appropriate views

acute fractures between the two approaches [2]. In both cases, fluoroscopic views should be used to localize the fracture and plan the incision in order to avoid an excessively long scar in a visible area.

The standard open approach involves an incision of variable length, usually 7–8 cm [3], centered over the fracture and planned approximately 1 cm below the clavicle as templated on fluoroscopy. The skin should be handled carefully, avoiding excessive retraction or cautery in this subcutaneous bone. After subcutaneous dissection, the platysma is released [1]. Beneath that, the supraclavicular nerves, which run perpendicular to the incision, are identified in the wound [1, 3]. Often there is a particularly prominent nerve in the lateral aspect of the incision. These nerves should be protected throughout the case, if possible, to avoid peri-incisional numbness. After this, the clavipectoral fascia along the clavicle should be incised [1], usually extending a rent through it made by the fracture. The fracture ends are identified and the bone exposed medially and laterally to make room for plate fixation. Small Hohmann retractors can be placed behind the clavicle to aid in exposure.

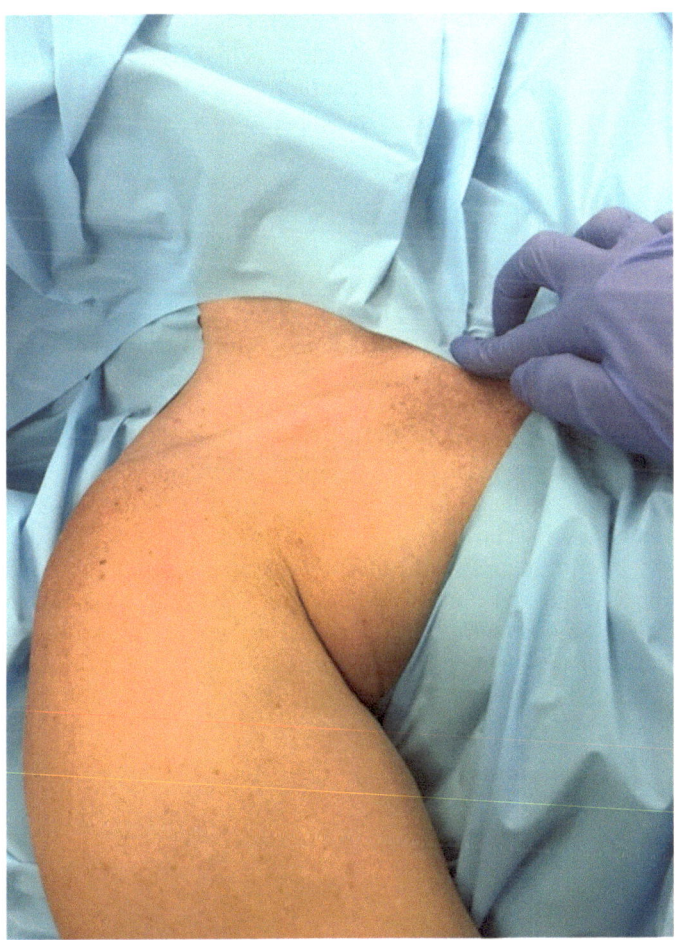

FIGURE 1.3 The clavicle must be exposed medially up to the sternal notch

In the MIPO approach [4], a 2–3 cm lateral incision is first made along the anterior border of the clavicle as localized by X-ray. The dissection proceeds between the trapezius and the deltoid muscles, and the clavicle is exposed by detaching the deltoid from the bone's superior surface. Following this, a tunnel is created from lateral to medial underneath the musculature with a periosteal elevator. Care is taken to keep the elevator along the bone, and avoid placement into the soft tissues near the vasculature and brachial plexus. A counter incision is then performed medially, and dissection proceeds in a lateral direction with the elevator in a similar fashion.

Reduction Techniques

The standard open approach exposes the fracture fragments directly. They can be reduced using clamps of the surgeon's choice, Kirschner wires (to hold butterfly fragments), or a mini-distractor [1] (Fig. 1.4). These clamps should not be placed deeply behind the bone to avoid injury to vessels and the brachial plexus [4]. The subclavian vein sits inferior to the clavicle, underneath the subclavius muscle, and the artery and brachial plexus are more posterior, deep to the anterior scalene muscle [1]. Regardless of plate position, these structures are approximately 8–12 mm away from the bone, and over-penetration of reduction tools, wires, or drills is ill-advised [5].

In the MIPO approach, the fracture is not exposed directly, and reduction is achieved primarily through fluoroscopic alignment [4]. K wires or 4.0 Schanz screws, placed out of the

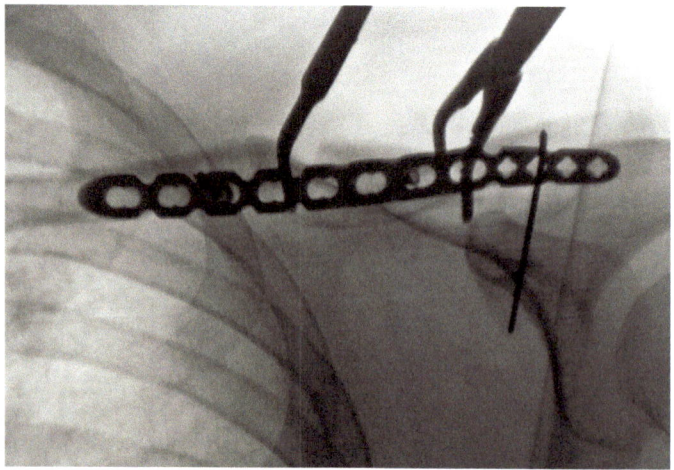

FIGURE 1.4 Reduction of a clavicle fracture using clamps

planned path of the plate, can be used as joysticks to align the fracture. One author recommends a 2 or 2.5 mm titanium elastic nail inserted medial to lateral as a temporary reduction tool [6]. The plate itself can also be used for reduction with attachment of screws laterally, followed by clamping of the plate to the medial fragment through the medial incision [4]. The screw placement sequence involves placing a locking drill bit into the most lateral plate hole, followed by a cortical screw in the third lateral hole to pull the plate to the bone. The locking drill bit should be pulled back slightly before screw tightening to avoid breakage. This is followed by a locking screw in the most lateral hole. The same process is repeated on the medial side [2, 4, 7].

Implant Choice

Regardless of plate choice, at least three screws on each side of the fracture should be used [4] to ensure a stable construct. Pre-contoured specialty plates (Fig. 1.5) fit most clavicles but not all, and the surgeon must be prepared to bend the plate if necessary. Many of these plates have a cluster of lateral locking holes, which provide good fixation in osteoporotic bone.

A 3.5 reconstruction or similar type plate, or multiple mini-fragment plates, will need to be contoured to fit the clavicle. In the direct approach, this is done in situ after the bone ends are reduced. In the MIPO approach, the curve of the unaffected clavicle on a caudal tilt X-ray [4] can be used as a template, or the plate can be bent prior to surgery using a sawbone clavicle. If a fluoroscopic templating approach is chosen, the plate bending proceeds lateral to medial [4]. For an anterior plate, the concave lateral bend is made first with a locking drill sleeve attached to the plate to avoid deforming the locking hole. This bend is aligned with the clavicle on fluoroscopy, and then the medial end is bent in a convex direction at the point where the clavicle begins to curve. For a superior plate, the contralateral clavicle is used as a template. The plate is flipped upside down, and the lateral and medial bends are made. This usually causes a deformation in the coronal plane and will require straightening [7].

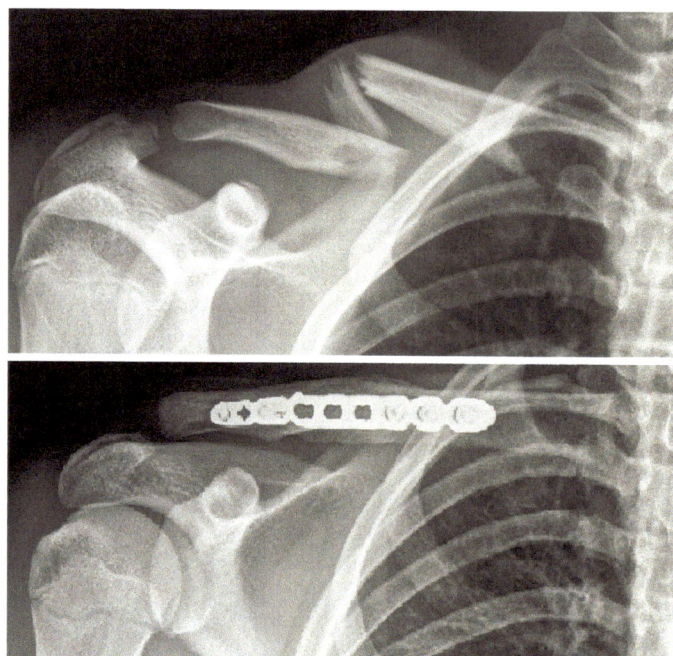

FIGURE 1.5 Pre-contoured plate used to treat a displaced fracture

Plate Placement

Studies disagree over which placement construct, anterior or superior, has greater biomechanical stability. One study shows no differences in union rates or outcomes between the two in the MIPO approach [7]. The advantages of anteroinferior plating (Fig. 1.6) include aiming the screws in a posterior-superior direction, away from the vessels [1], less implant prominence, and the ability to place longer screws to improve purchase in the lateral clavicle. The superior plate (Fig. 1.7), on the other hand, has limited fixation in the lateral clavicle due to the thin bone in the superior-inferior direction.

The double-plate construct (Fig. 1.8) is a relatively new method of plate fixation [3]. It is based on the idea that the natural motion of the clavicle is in multiple planes, and

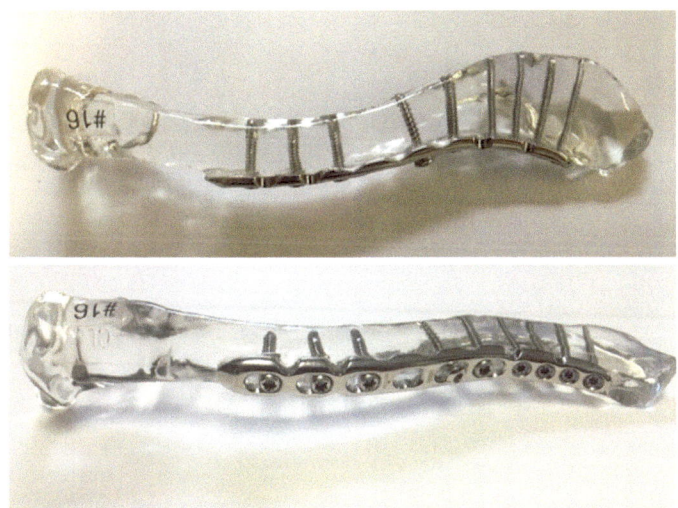

FIGURE 1.6 Anterior clavicle plate

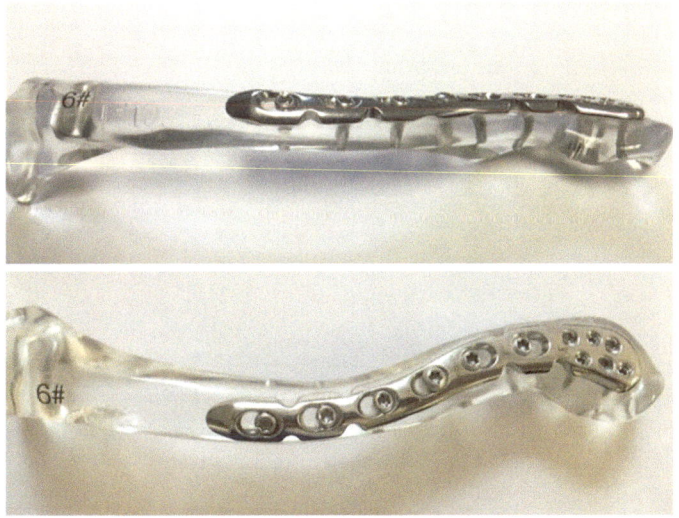

FIGURE 1.7 Superior clavicle plate

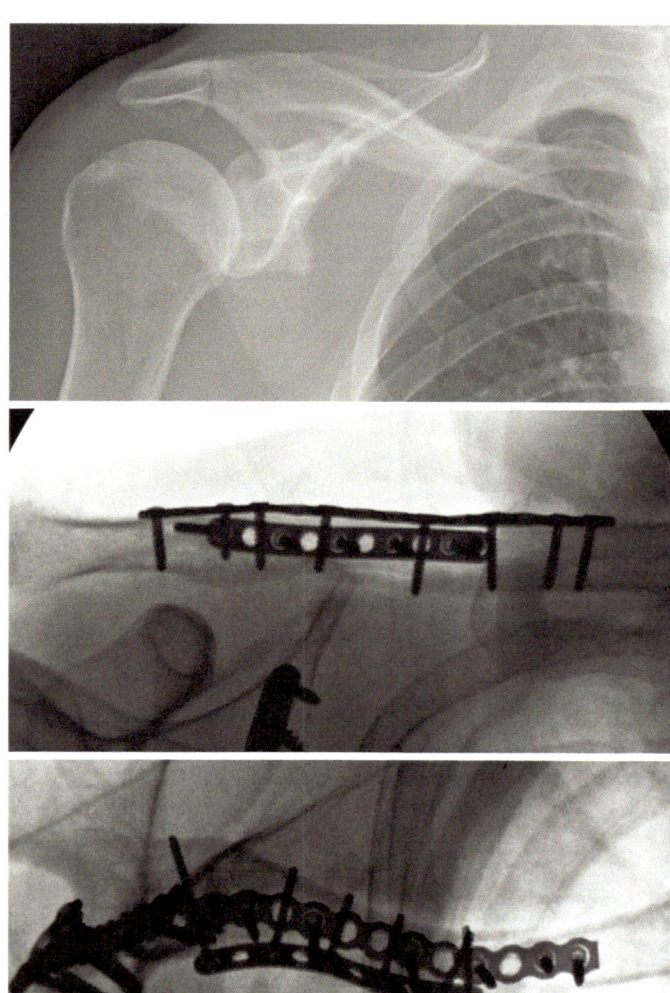

FIGURE 1.8 Double plating method used to treat a displaced fracture. Scapular plates are also seen intraoperatively

therefore multiple planes of fixation are beneficial. It involves a standard open approach with a 2.4 mm locking compression plate placed anteriorly and a slightly longer 2.7

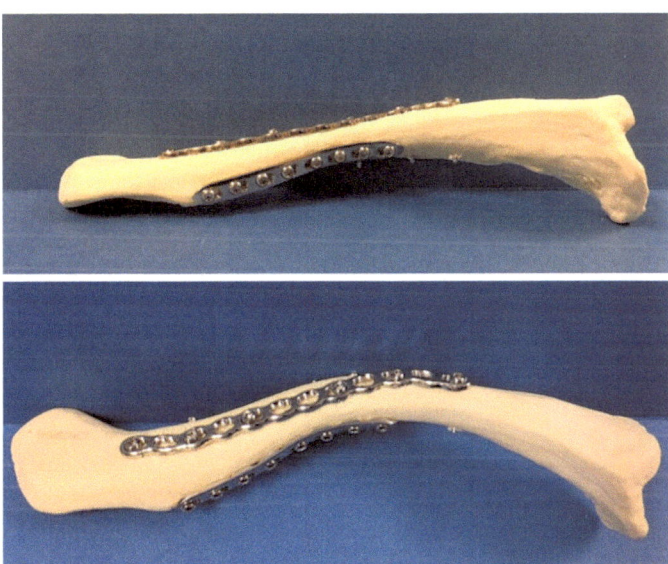

FIGURE 1.9 Double plate construct with the plates bent to the shape of the clavicle

reconstruction plate placed superiorly (Fig. 1.9). The fracture pattern dictates which plate is fixed to the bone first. In at least one study, this construct was superior to the 3.5 reconstruction plate in multiplanar stiffness [3]. The smaller, low-profile plates may also decrease the need for implant removal.

Closure

Deep closure should be limited to bringing the clavipectoral fascia to cover the plate. The supraclavicular nerves should remain protected and not tied tightly into the closure. Subcutaneous suture is then performed, followed by the skin. Suture choice is dependent on the surgeon and should strive to minimize scar formation.

References

1. Collinge C, Devinney S, Herscovici D, et al. Anterior-inferior plate fixation of middle-third fractures and nonunions of the clavicle. J Orthop Trauma. 2006;20(10):680–6.
2. Sohn HS, Kim WJ, Shon MS. Comparison between open plating versus minimally invasive plate osteosynthesis for acute displaced clavicular shaft fractures. Injury. 2015;46(8):1577–84.
3. Prasarn ML, Meyers KN, Wilkin G, et al. Dual mini-fragment plating for midshaft clavicle fractures: a clinical and biomechanical investigation. Arch Orthop Trauma Surg. 2015;135:1655–62.
4. Sohn HS, Kim BY, Shin SJ. A surgical technique for minimally invasive plate osteosynthesis of clavicular midshaft fractures. J Orthop Trauma. 2013;27(4):e92–6.
5. Hussey MM, Chen Y, Fajardo RA, et al. Analysis of neurovascular safety between superior and anterior plating techniques of clavicle fractures. J Orthop Trauma. 2013;27(11):627–32.
6. Lee HJ, Oh CW, Oh JK, et al. Percutaneous plating for comminuted midshaft fractures of the clavicle: a surgical technique to aid the reduction with nail assistance. Injury. 2013;44(4):465–70.
7. Sohn HS, Shon MS, Lee KH, et al. Clinical comparison of two different plating methods in minimally invasive plate osteosynthesis for clavicular midshaft fractures: a randomized controlled trial. Injury. 2015;46(11):2230–8.

Chapter 2
Acromioclavicular and Sternoclavicular Joint Injuries

Mark Dunleavy and Damian M. Rispoli

Sternoclavicular Injuries

Statistics and Introduction

The most often cited incidence of sternoclavicular (SC) injuries is less than 3% of all injuries to the shoulder girdle from 1958 [1]. They are uncommon injuries often associated with high energy. Fractures of the medial aspect of the clavicle can also present challenges with respect to safe exposure and fixation. Bipolar injuries affecting both ends of the clavicle can present complicated and daunting challenges. Anterior dislocations present more commonly than posterior dislocations and can often be treated non-operatively.

M. Dunleavy
Penn State Health Milton S. Hershey Medical Center,
Hershey, PA, USA

D. M. Rispoli (✉)
Musculoskeletal Institute, Geisinger Health System,
Lemoyne, PA, USA
e-mail: drispoli@geisinger.edu

© Springer Nature Switzerland AG 2020   13
D. S. Horwitz et al. (eds.), *Tips and Tricks for Problem Fractures, Volume I*,
https://doi.org/10.1007/978-3-030-38274-2_2

Anatomy

Any motion of the shoulder results in movement at the SC joint. The clavicle rotates up to 40° along its longitudinal axis [2]. The clavicle is the first long bone to ossify (intrauterine week 5) and the last to fuse at its medial epiphysis (average 23–25 years of age with reports of delayed closure up to age 31) [3]. The medial clavicle provides the bony attachment sites of the clavicular head of the pectoralis major on its anterior surface, the sternocleidomastoid on its posterior surface and the sternohyoid on its inferior posterior surface. Inferiorly, there is a 2 cm roughened area for the attachment of the costoclavicular ligaments.

The ligaments that comprise the soft tissue restraint of the SC joint are the capsular ligament which attaches predominantly to the medial physis (strongest) [4, 5] intra-articular disc (checkrein to medial displacement), costoclavicular ligaments (single most important constraint to SC motion) [6], and the interclavicular ligament (superior constraint) [7].

Posterior dislocation of the SC joint has the possibility of causing serious injury to the hilar structures. There are multiple reports in the literature of damage to the great vessels (trachea, esophagus, anterior neck vasculature, and brachial plexus). Clinical findings of hoarseness, dysphagia, or dyspnea should always prompt further clinical and radiographic evaluation. Unreduced posterior dislocations have been associated with thoracic outlet syndrome, vascular compromise, compression of the trachea and esophagus, and the risk of erosion into vital posterior structures. Despite these dire risks, few deaths have been reported in the literature because of posterior SC dislocations [8].

Imaging

Plain radiographs of the SC joint are often time difficult to obtain and image quality can be less than satisfactory. The most accepted radiographic views are Serendipity view, a 40°

cephalic tilt view [5], and Hobbs view (posterior to anterior with the neck parallel to the cassette) [9]. A computed tomography (CT) scan with or without three-dimensional (3D) reconstruction is the imaging study of choice for evaluation of the SC joint. On typical presentation in a polytrauma patient, determination of the presence or direction of dislocation is quite challenging, making the CT scan an indispensable tool.

Classification

Simply defined with the direction of the dislocation.

Options

Anterior Sternoclavicular Dislocation

The current literature supports the non-operative treatment of anterior sternoclavicular dislocations (69% good/excellent results) [10]. Surgical repair of the SC ligaments should be considered with unstable anterior dislocations in the presence of fracture requiring fixation. Suture material placed in the capsular ligaments may be fixated to the plate through drill holes in the clavicle or utilizing anchors in the medial clavicle.

Posterior Sternoclavicular Dislocation

Posterior SC dislocations should be treated with closed reduction with open reduction and fixation considered for unstable or irreducible dislocations. Closed reduction and open reduction yields good/excellent results in 96% [11].

Preferred Surgical Technique

Patient Positioning

Patient placed supine on the operating table.

A bump should be placed in the midline between the scapulae. The bump should allow for the shoulders to just comfortably lie on the surgical table surface.

The affected shoulder should be just at or extending over the table's edge to allow for maximal exposure.

The upper extremity of the affected side should be draped free and the contralateral shoulder should be palpable to apply counter-traction or stabilize the patient on the surgical table while traction is applied to the affected side.

It has been suggested that a folded sheet can be placed around the patient's thorax in case counter-traction is needed to counteract the traction on the affected side.

Care should be taken to drape and thus allow for appropriate cardiothoracic intervention in the unlikely event the assistance of a thoracic surgeon is required.

Closed Reduction

Overriding Principle – distraction of the SC joint with anterior translation to reduce the joint.

- Abduction: Laterally directed force with the shoulder abducted. Progressive extension of the shoulder.
- Adduction: Traction applied to the adducted shoulder with concomitant downward pressure.

A pointed towel clamp around the medial shaft of the clavicle or grasping the bone can be helpful to add a focused anterior translation to the medial clavicle.

Approach

An anterior incision is used that parallels the superior border of the medial 3–4 inches of the clavicle.

The incision extends downward over the sternum just medial to the involved SC joint.

It is important to remove sufficient soft tissue to expose the joint but to still leave the anterior capsular ligament intact.

Procedure

The medial clavicle should then be reduced back to its articulation with the manubrium.

Suture repair of the anterior ligaments to grossly stabilize the SC joint with the goal of preventing recurrent posterior dislocation has been performed utilizing local or allograft tissue [11–14], plate or screw fixation [15, 16], or suture anchor stabilization [17]. Successful medial clavicular resection and ligament reconstruction have been noted to be successful [18–21]. Stabilization without bony resection is the preference of the senior author.

Post-operatively

Patients should be placed in a figure-of eight dressing to hold the shoulders back for 4–6 weeks to allow for healing of the soft tissues.

Pearls and Pitfalls

Use of K-wires, Steinmann pins, and smooth pins should be avoided given their documented propensity toward migration with untoward results [22].

The low numbers of reported outcomes from open reduction and fixation do not allow for differentiation between the various methods [10].

The most important factor affecting outcomes is time since injury; therefore, prompt diagnosis and treatment is optimal [10].

Acromioclavicular Injuries

Statistics and Introduction

Acromioclavicular (AC) joint injuries are reported to have an incidence of 1.5–1.8 per 100,000 inhabitants per year, male:female ratio of 8.5:1, just over 50% occurring from age 20 to 39, and the two most common etiologies were sports (#1, cycling and contact sports) and motor vehicle collisions (#2) [23, 24]. Fractures of the lateral aspect of the clavicle can also present challenges for acromioclavicular joint repair with respect to reconstruction, repair, and fixation.

Anatomy

The clavicle rotates up to 40° along its longitudinal axis [2]. However, due to synchronous scapuloclavicular motion there is only 5°–8° of rotation at the AC joint [25].

- Static stabilizers: AC joint capsule (posterosuperior ligaments – posterior translation) and the posterior and superior AC ligaments (horizontal motion) [26]. Coracoclavicular (CC) ligaments (conoid greater than trapezoid) as restraint to vertical translation [27].
- Dynamic stabilizers: Origin of the anterior deltoid and the insertion of the trapezius muscle [28].

Imaging

Routine radiographs include true anterior-posterior and axillary lateral of the shoulder along with Zanca views (10°–15° degree cephalic tilt) [29]. Radiographs should be obtained in an upright position with the arm unsupported. A combined view including both acromioclavicular joints can be helpful for grading/classifying the injury and for surgical planning. A CT scan with or without 3D reconstruction can be of

significant benefit in fractures with associated acromioclavicular joint disruption.

Classification [30]

- Type I: AC ligaments and the joint remain stable
- Type II: AC ligaments are ruptured (horizontal instability);
  CC ligament remains intact (vertically stable)
- Type III: AC and CC ligaments are torn, resulting in com-
  plete AC dislocation
- Type IV: AC and CC ligaments are torn and the distal end
  of the clavicle posteriorly dislocates
- Type V: More severe version of a Type III injury (3 × nor-
  mal CC distance).
- Type VI: Inferior displacement of the clavicle

Options [31]

Types I and II are universally treated non-operatively. Type
III is controversial with most authors considering fixation in
young active individuals. Types IV–VI are treated
operatively.

While measurement of the coracoclavicular distance may
be beneficial in differentiating between types II and III, the
senior author prefers to have the patients perform cross-arm
abduction with the shoulder at 90° of elevation/abduction. If
the lateral clavicle overrides the acromion, the injury is
grossly unstable and should be operatively fixed.

Patient Positioning

Beach chair configuration
   A small roll may be placed under the ipsilateral scapula to
bring the shoulder forward (this allows good access to the
superior aspect of the shoulder).

Ensure proper placement of the fluoroscopy equipment to allow for intraoperative imaging.

It is beneficial to prep the arm free to allow for manipulation of the arm and application of traction during surgery.

Open Approach

Saber type skin incision 2–3 cm medial to the AC joint 6–10 cm.

Full-thickness subcutaneous flaps are developed medially and laterally

Incise the periosteum and reflect the deltotrapezius fascia in a medial to lateral direction at the junction of the anterior and middle third of the clavicle.

Subperiosteal exposure of the lateral clavicle keeping the flaps continuous with the deltotrapezial fascia.

Split the fibers of the deltoid anteriorly to expose the medial and lateral aspect of the coracoid base.

Fixation

The overriding principle should be to place the torn ends of the CC ligaments together and hold them in this position for at least 6 consecutive weeks.

Currently acceptable options include Hook plate (Balser) [32], screw fixation (Bosworth) [33], suture fixation (multiple authors), and ligament reconstruction (Weaver-Dunn, Jones, Mazocca) [34–36]. These techniques may be open, arthroscopic, or a combination of both.

Tips and Tricks

Utilize a technique that you are comfortable and trained to perform. For most orthopaedic trauma surgeons, this involves an open procedure. Hook plates can be difficult to accurately place and require a second operation to remove the fixation but can give a satisfying and stable reduction. An open procedure using suture fixation can be a safe and straight forward method of fixation. Remember to keep bone bridges in the clavicle as wide as possible to avoid stress risers and intra- or post-operative fractures. Key your fixation of the clavicle to the coracoid off the reduced acromioclavicular joint. Use temporary K-wire cross fixation of the AC joint to hold reduction and ensure proper alignment of the clavicle and scapula. Expose the base of the coracoid by placing Homan retractors medially and laterally to ensure solid fixation and/or safe passage of grafts or suture.

References

1. Cave EF, editor. Fractures and other injuries. Year Book Publishers: Chicago; 1958.
2. Sewell MD, Al-Hadithy N, Le Leu A, Lambert SM. Instability of the sternoclavicular joint: current concepts in classification, treatment and outcomes. Bone Joint J. 2013;95-B:721–31.
3. Webb PA, Suchey JM. Epiphyseal union of the anterior iliac crest and medial clavicle in a modern multiracial sample of American males and females. Am J Phys Anthropol. 1985;68(4):457–66.
4. Bearn JG. Direct observations on the function of the capsule of the sternoclavicular joint in clavicular support. J Anat. 1967;101:159–70.
5. Rockwood CA Jr. Disorders of the sternoclavicular joint. In: Rockwood Jr CA, Matsen FA, editors. The shoulder. Philadelphia: WB Saunders; 1990. p. 477–525.
6. Kapanjii I. The physiology of joints, vol. 1. Baltimore: Williams & Wilkins; 1970.
7. Basamajian JV, Bazant FJ. Factors preventing downward displacement of the adducted shoulder joint. J Bone Joint Surg. 1959;41A:1182.
8. Miller MD, Rispoli DM. Sternoclavicular disorders in Shoulder Surgery: An Illustrated Textbook. In: Wulker N, Mansat M, Fu FH, editors. Shoulder Surgery: An Illustrated Textbook. London: Martin Duntz; 2001. p. 451–461.
9. Hobbs DW. Sternoclavicular joint: a new axial radiographic view. Radiology. 1968;90:801–2.

10. Glass ER, Thompson JD, Cole PA, Gause TM, Altman GT. Treatment of sternoclavicular joint dislocations: a systematic review of 251 dislocations in 24 case series. J Trauma. 2011;70(5):1294–8.

11. Pearsall AW, Russel GV. Ipsilateral clavicle fracture, sternoclavicular joint subluxation, and long thoracic nerve injury: an unusual constellation of injuries sustained during wrestling. AJ Sports Med. 2000;28(6):904–8.

12. Burri C, Neugebauer R. Carbon fiber replacement of the ligaments of the shoulder girdle and the treatment of lateral instability of the ankle joint. Clin Orthop. 1985;196:112–7.

13. Bisson LJ, Dauphin N, Marzo JM. A safe zone for resection of the medial end of the clavicle. J Shoulder Elb Surg. 2003;12(6):592–4.

14. Armstrong AL, Dias JJ. Reconstruction for instability of the sternoclavicular joint using the tendon of the sternocleidomastoid muscle. J Bone Joint Surg Br. 2008;90:610–3.

15. Fery A, Leonard A. Transsternal sternoclavicular projection: diagnostic value in sternoclavicular dislocations. J Radiol. 1981;62:167–70.

16. Brinkler MR, Bartz RL, Reardon PR, et al. A method for open reduction and internal fixation of the unstable posterior sternoclavicular joint dislocation. J Orthop Trauma. 1997;11:378–81.

17. Abiddin Z, Sinopidis C, Grocock CJ, et al. Suture anchors for treatment of sternoclavicular joint instability. J Shoulder Elb Surg. 2006;15:315–8.

18. Porral MA. Observation d'une double luxation de la clavicule droite. J Univ Hebd Med Chir Prat. 1831;2:78–82.

19. Dutta AK, Wirth MA, Rockwood CA Jr. Sternoclavicular joint injuries. Rockwood and Green's fractures in adults. Philadelphia: Lippincott Williams & Wilkins; 2001. p. 1243–75.

20. Marker LB, Klareskov B. Posterior sternoclavicular dislocation: an American football injury. Br J Sports Med. 1996;30(1):71–2.

21. Bicos J, Nicholson GP. Treatment and results of sternoclavicular injuries. Clin Sports Med. 2003;22:359–70.

22. Lyons FA, Rockwood CA. Migration of pins used in operations on the shoulder. J Bone Joint Surg. 1990;72:1262–7.

23. Nordqvist A, Petersson CJ. Incidence and causes of shoulder girdle injuries in an urban population. J Shoulder Elb Surg. 1995;4(2):107–12.

24. Chillemi C, Franceschini V, Dei Giudici L, et al. Epidemiology of isolated acromioclavicular joint dislocation. Emerg Med Int. 2013;2013:171609. https://doi.org/10.1155/2013/171609. Epub 2013 Jan 28

25. Flatow EL. The biomechanics of the acromioclavicular, sternoclavicular, and scapulothoracic joints. Instr Course Lect. 1993;42:237–45.

26. Klimkiewicz JJ, Williams GR, Sher JS, Karduna A, Des Jardins J, Ianotti JP. The acromioclavicular capsule as a restraint to posterior translation of the clavicle: a biomechanical analysis. J Shoulder Elb Surg. 1999;8:119–24.

27. Fukuda K, Caig EV, An KN, Cofield RH, Chao EY. Biomechanical study of the ligamentous system of the acromioclavicular joint. J Bone Joint Surg. 1986;8A:119–24.

28. Lizaur A, Marco L, Cebrian R. Acute dislocation of the acromioclavicular joint: traumatic anatomy and the importance of the deltoid and trapezius. J Bone Joint Surg. 1994;76:602–6.

29. Zanca P. Shoulder pain: involvement of the acromioclavicular joint (analysis of 1,000 cases). Am J Roentgenol Radium Ther Nucl Med. 1971;112(3):493–506.

30. Rockwood CA, Green DP. Fractures in adults, vol. 860. Philadelphia: Lippincott-Raven; 1984.

31. Simovitch R, Sanders B, Ozbaydar M, Lavery K, Warner JJP. Acromioclavicular joint injuries: diagnosis and management. J Am Acad Orthop Surg. 2009 Apr;17(4):207–19.

32. Balser D. Eine neue. Moethode zur operativve Behandlung der akromioklavikularen luxation. Chir Prax. 1976;24:275.

33. Bosworth BM. Acromioclavicular separation: a new method of repair. Surg Gynecol Obstet. 1941;73:866–71.

34. Weave JK, Dunn HK. Treartment of acromioclavicular injuries, especially complete acromioclavicular separation. J Bone Joint Surg. 1972;54A:1187–94.

35. Jones HP, Lemos MJ, Schepsis AA. Salvage of failed acromioclavicular joint reconstruction using autogenous semitendinosus tendon from the knee: surgical technique and case report. Am J Sports Med. 2001;21:1277.

36. Mazzocca AD, Santangelo SA, Johnson ST, Dumonski ML, Arciero RA. A biomechanical evaluation of an anatomical coracoclavicular ligament reconstruction. Am J Sports Med. 2006;34:236–46.

Chapter 3
Proximal Humerus Fractures

Jaclyn M. Jankowski, Richard S. Yoon, and Frank A. Liporace

Introduction

Currently, proximal humerus fractures make up 7% of all fractures and 80% of all humerus fractures. In patients older than 65, proximal humerus fractures make up more than 10% of all fractures and are the third most common non-vertebral osteoporotic fracture following fractures of the distal radius and proximal femur [1]. There are a variety of treatment options for proximal humerus fractures, including non-operative management, percutaneous pinning, screw osteosynthesis, plating, intramedullary nailing, and arthroplasty (hemi, total, and reverse) [2]. According to Hasty et al., 85% of fractures between 2005 and 2012 were treated

J. M. Jankowski
Department of Orthopaedic Surgery, Jersey City Medical Center – RWJ Barnabas Health, Jersey City, NJ, USA

R. S. Yoon · F. A. Liporace (✉)
Division of Orthopaedic Trauma and Adult Reconstruction, Department of Orthopaedic Surgery, Jersey City Medical Center – RWJ Barnabas Health, Jersey City, NJ, USA

© Springer Nature Switzerland AG 2020   25
D. S. Horwitz et al. (eds.), *Tips and Tricks for Problem Fractures, Volume I*,
https://doi.org/10.1007/978-3-030-38274-2_3

non-operatively, but rates of operative management have significantly increased over that same period of time for all fracture types [3].

Our preferred method of operative management is open reduction internal fixation (ORIF) with a locked plate construct. The main advantages of locked plating are the ability to use the plate as an indirect reduction technique and the potential for short immobilization and early range of motion due to the high initial stability that can be achieved [4]. Clinically, ORIF shows trends towards greater post-operative range of motion when compared to non-operative management [5]. The only significant difference in complications between operative and non-operative management is the rate of reoperation [6].

Prior studies have shown a 36% complication rate with ORIF but improved hardware and appropriate technique can mitigate and minimize these complications. For example, using a combination of convergent and divergent head screws increases pullout strength, and ensuring that screws are the appropriate length and are placed in the strong subchondral bone of the head can prevent cutout. Additionally, locked plates have decreased stiffness compared to non-locked plates, which allow them to withstand increased cyclic loading [2, 7]. If anatomic reduction is achieved and appropriate fixation techniques are utilized, ORIF can have good long-term results. Here, we review our preferred approach and provide case examples in which we use it.

Authors' Preferred Approach: General Principles and Case Examples

Our preferred approach to fixing proximal humerus fractures is the deltopectoral approach. While the deltoid split is also a viable option, as it arguably makes hardware placement easier, it does not allow for visualization of the more anterior bony and soft tissue landmarks that can often assist in obtaining desired reconstruction. Overall, through the deltopectoral interval, fixing proximal humerus fractures can be reliably performed via a stepwise approach, regardless of fracture pattern. This stepwise approach consists of the following:

1. Adequate exposure and bursectomy
2. Tagging the greater and lesser tuberosities with non-absorbable suture
3. Provisional reduction and fixation of the plate to the proximal fragment
4. Non-locking fixation of the plate to the shaft, which restores valgus
5. Reinforcing fixation of tuberosities to the plate

In general, following this stepwise method can allow for reliable, efficient reduction and fixation of proximal humerus fractures, regardless of fracture type. Our table preference is to perform the surgery on a beach chair, turned orthogonal with anesthesia, allowing imaging to come in from behind the patient. It is important to ensure that the endotracheal tube is facing the contralateral direction and one must use caution not to drape oneself out of the wound (you must be able to palpate the coracoid). Also, take note of any cardiac leads that may be in the way of imaging and ask anesthesia to move them accordingly. On the approach, the cephalic vein should be mobilized in the direction that it seems to favor, the subdeltoid space cleared bluntly, and the biceps tendon within the bicipital groove, which acts as a notable landmark for future plate placement. It is important to note that, especially in the elderly population, if the biceps tendon is damaged or chronically inflamed-appearing, an in situ pectoral tenodesis is performed. Clearing the hemarthrosis and bursal space is of utmost importance in order to identify the greater and lesser tuberosities for tagging with non-absorbable suture. Here the suture can be utilized as reduction aids in order to reconstruct the tuberosities with the head. With exposure achieved and suture placed and provisional reduction able to be achieved, the next step is plate fixation. Next, we review specific case examples exhibiting fixation sequence and strategies to obtain your desired outcome.

Case 1: Avoiding Varus

The patient is a 64-year-old female status post-fall from standing height. Patient sustained a right proximal humerus fracture (Figs. 3.1 and 3.2). Imaging analysis exhibited a large greater tuberosity fragment along with a separate lesser tuberosity fragment noted on computed tomography (CT) (Figs. 3.1 and 3.2). Here, heavy, non-absorbable sutures were used to tag and reapproximate the greater and lesser tuberosities, which were in close enough proximity to fix the proximal portion of the plate to head-tuberosities with Kirschner (K) wires (Fig. 3.3). Imaging confirmed appropriate plate height, and K wires were exchanged with locking screws with the plate still off of the shaft distally; fixing the proximal portion first allows for non-locking screw placement in the shaft, which will restore valgus (Fig. 3.4). Plate position is again checked and then the remaining screws filled in the head and shaft (Fig. 3.5). Once final fixation is complete, it is important to get multiple views (we prefer to

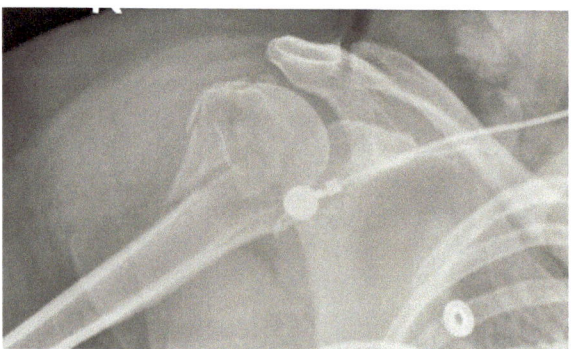

FIGURE 3.1 A 64-year-old female following a fall, here, an anteroposterior (AP) radiograph exhibiting a proximal humerus fracture with a large greater tuberosity fragment

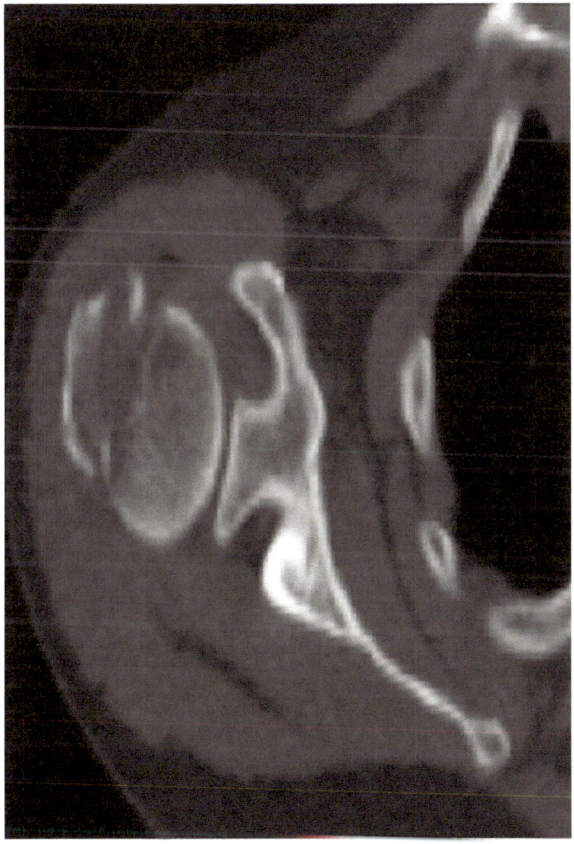

FIGURE 3.2 Axial CT imaging here, noted a separate lesser tuberosity fragment that was not readily obvious on plain radiographs

perform live fluoroscopy) to ensure that screw lengths are appropriate (Fig. 3.6). Reproducing this stepwise approach has offered efficient, reliable results for the majority of operative proximal humerus fractures.

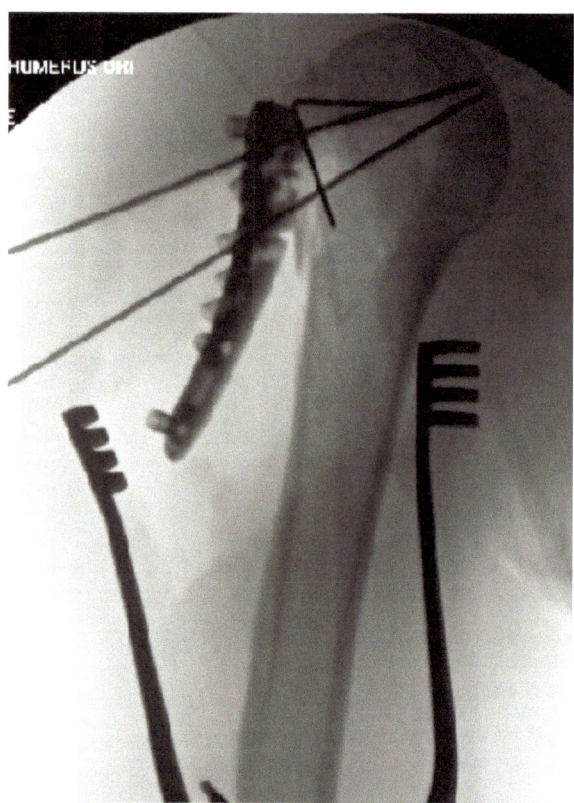

FIGURE 3.3 Following adequate exposure through the deltopectoral interval fixation of the tuberosities with non-absorbable sutures allows for provisional reduction and proximal plate fixation. Here, exaggerated positioning of the plate is desired

Case 2: Avoiding Impingement

A 34-year-old right-hand-dominant male sustained a closed, right proximal humerus fracture status post-fall down the stairs. Radiographs exhibited a proximal humerus fracture

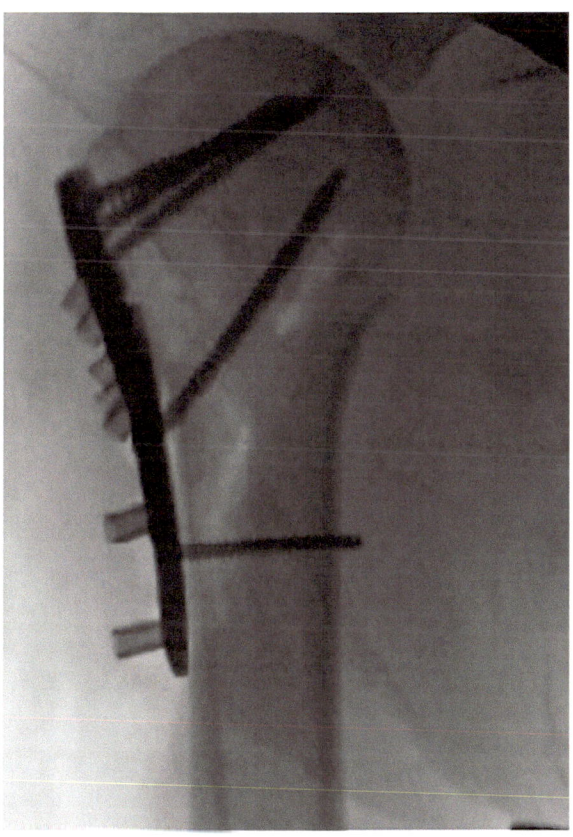

FIGURE 3.4 The exaggerated plate position allows one to achieve further valgus once a non-locking shaft screw is placed

with a notable greater tuberosity fragment that was impacted and exhibited significant lateral prominence (Fig. 3.7). Advanced imaging via CT was performed and further delineated a tuberosity fragment that was "high-riding," thus increasing the chance of impingement if treated non-operatively (Fig. 3.8).

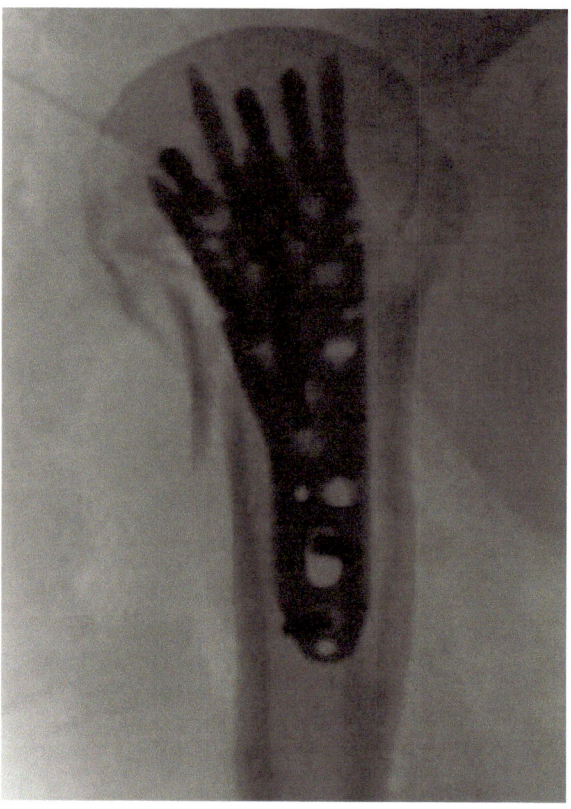

FIGURE 3.5 Prior to completely filling in with screws, ensure there is appropriate reduction and plate placement on the lateral view

This case is an important example of a fracture pattern that, if gone unrecognized, can do extremely poorly with non-operative treatment. Especially in a young person, reconstructing the greater tuberosity is essential to returning to overhead activities and avoiding impingement. Through the deltopectoral interval, our stepwise approach was applied; locked fixation into the head, followed by a non-

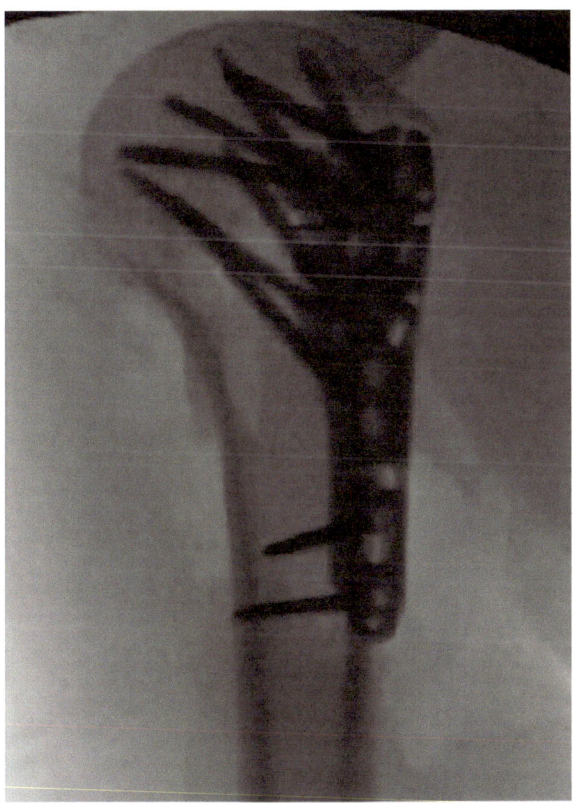

FIGURE 3.6 Remember, once the construct is complete, it is important to use live fluoroscopic imaging to ensure appropriate screw lengths

locking screw in the shaft (Fig. 3.9), ensuring the plate is correctly positioned over a well-reduced fracture on the lateral (Fig. 3.10), completing the construct by filling in locked screws and an additional non-locking screw in the shaft (Fig. 3.11) and, finally, using live fluoroscopy to ensure that

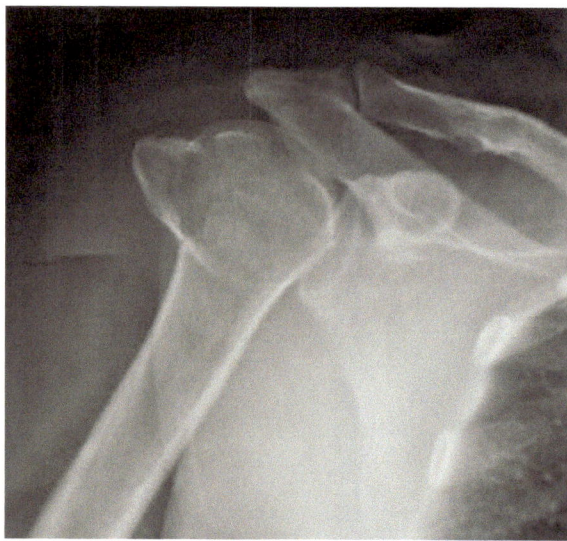

FIGURE 3.7 AP radiograph of a 34-year-old man exhibiting a right proximal humerus fracture with an impacted, lateral protruding greater tuberosity fragment

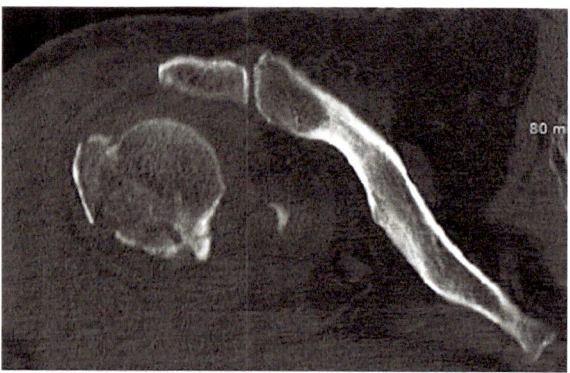

FIGURE 3.8 Coronal CT cut exhibiting a "high-riding," impacted greater tuberosity, increasing risk for impingement, especially when combined with the lateral protrusion

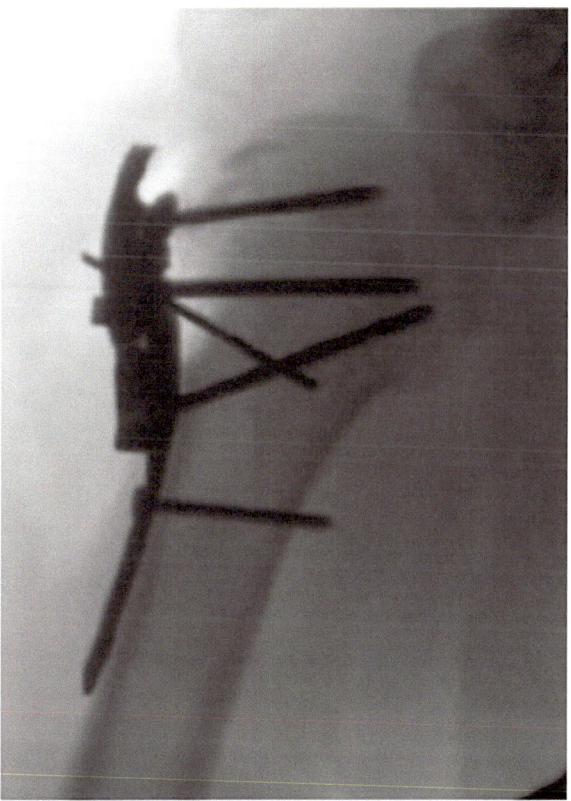

FIGURE 3.9 Following our systematic approach, suturing the tuberosities (following disimpaction of the greater) allows for reduction, proximal fixation followed by shaft screws to prevent varus

screw lengths are appropriate (Fig. 3.12). As another reminder, it is important to reinforce your tuberosity fixation by placing non-absorbable sutures through the plate to prevent further displacement, which can even be evident at final healing (Fig. 3.13).

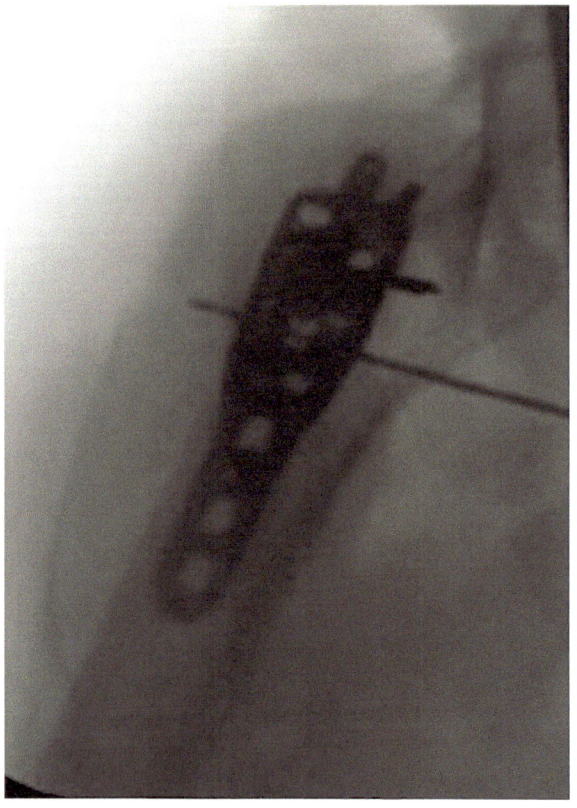

FIGURE 3.10 Follow the same steps, and check a lateral fluoroscopic image to ensure plate placement

Case 3: Supplemental Fixation

As is the case with any fracture, goals of fixation include creating a stable, reliable construct that allows for confident, early range of motion. Here, a 52-year-old right-hand-dominant male sustained a right proximal humerus fracture with a very large greater tuberosity fragment that seemed to extend posteriorly into the shaft (Fig. 3.14). Advanced imaging provided additional

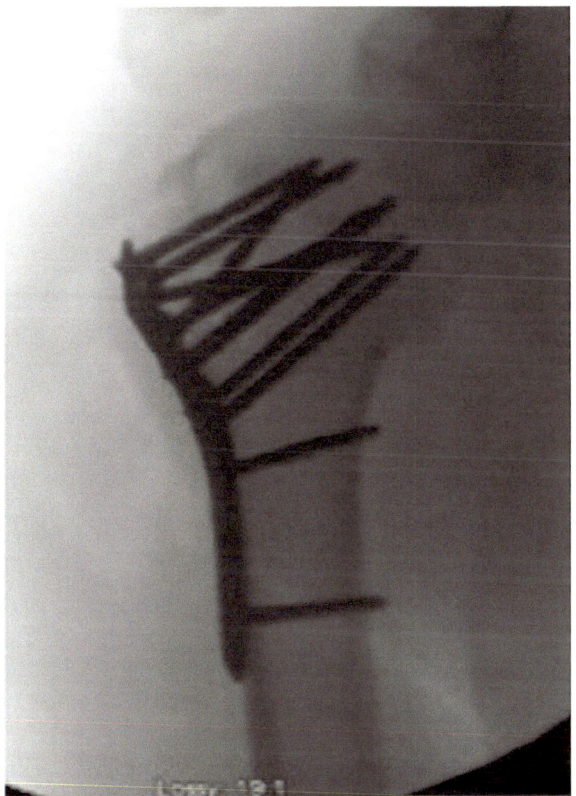

FIGURE 3.11 When satisfied, complete your fixation

information, exhibiting an impacted head (Fig. 3.15) along with a fracture in the coronal plane, which was the distal extension of the greater tuberosity piece (Fig. 3.16).

Following our stepwise approach, length, alignment, and rotation were restored (Fig. 3.17). However, initially, the coronal fracture line was not addressed and was found to be gapping during intraoperative range of motion, despite additional suture fixation. Therefore, in order to prevent gapping, the fracture was clamped, held provisionally with a K wire, and then a 3.5 mm reconstruction plate was placed on the posteroinferior aspect of the greater tuberosity, providing

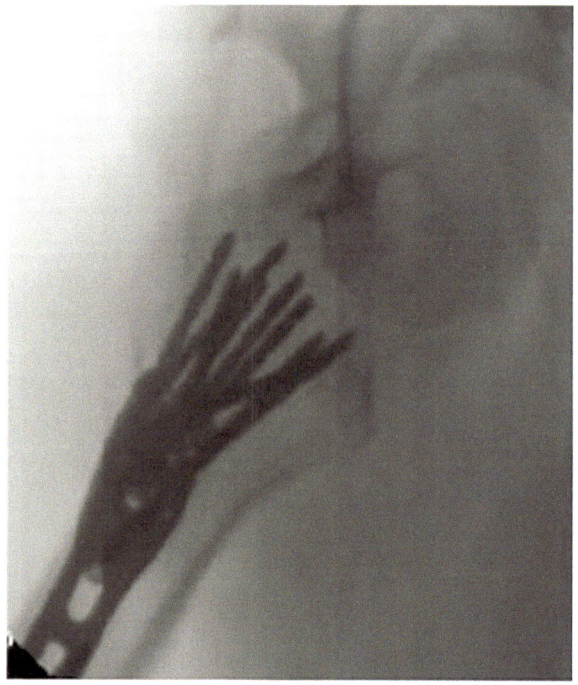

FIGURE 3.12 Remember, the last step is to use live fluoroscopy to ensure appropriate screw lengths

supplemental fixation (Figs. 3.18 and 3.19). Coronal fracture line gapping no longer occurred and the patient healed uneventfully with range of motion nearly restored and symmetric to his uninjured side at the 1-year follow-up time point (Figs. 3.20 and 3.21).

Summary

In summary, fixation of proximal humerus fractures, while challenging, can be made more facile by application of a systematic approach that follows the principles of obtaining

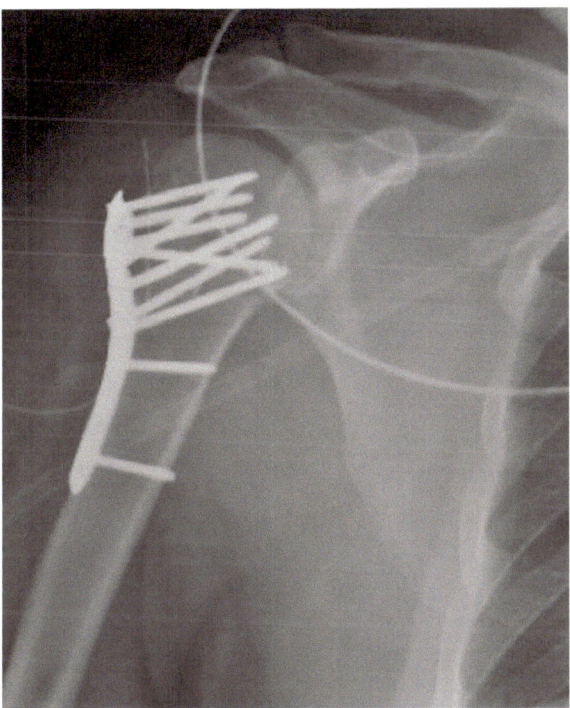

FIGURE 3.13 Final follow-up radiograph, exhibiting healed fractures. Note the importance of suture fixation back-up for the tuberosity fragments that prevented further posterosuperior escape

appropriate exposure, suture fixation/mobilization of the tuberosity fragments, and sequential reduction via proximal fixation followed by a non-locking shaft screw to remove varus. Additional tricks, as described by the cases above, can further add to one's arsenal in achieving stable, reliable fixation, allowing for early range of motion and an excellent functional outcome.

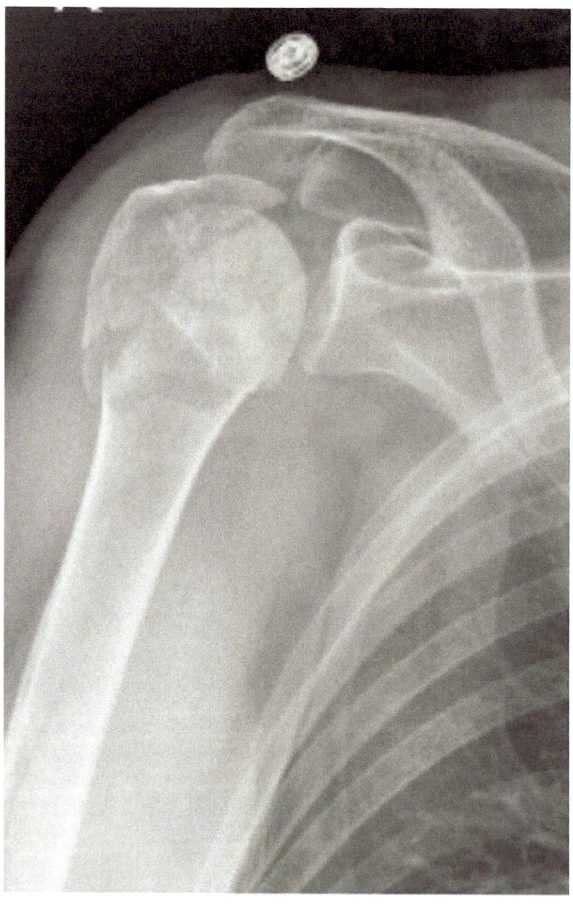

FIGURE 3.14 AP radiograph exhibiting a large greater tuberosity fragment with seemingly distal extension of the fracture line posteriorly

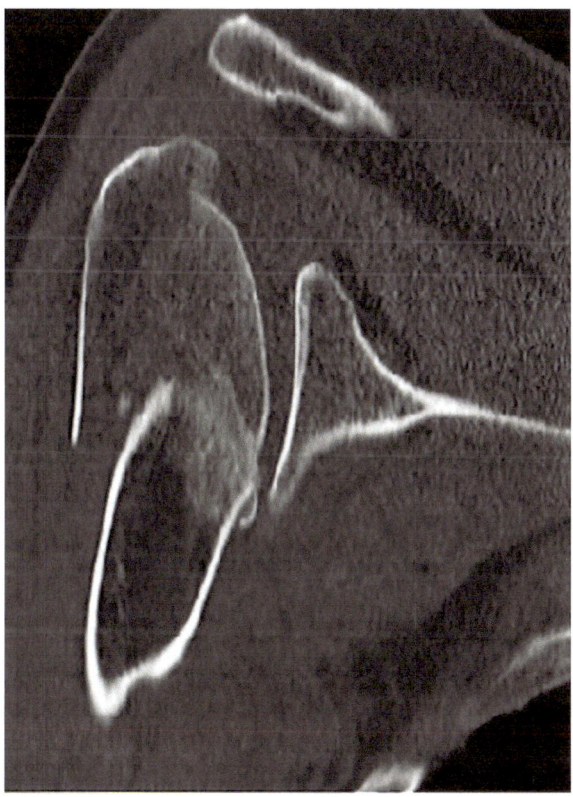

FIGURE 3.15 CT coronal cut showing an impacted head fragment into the shaft

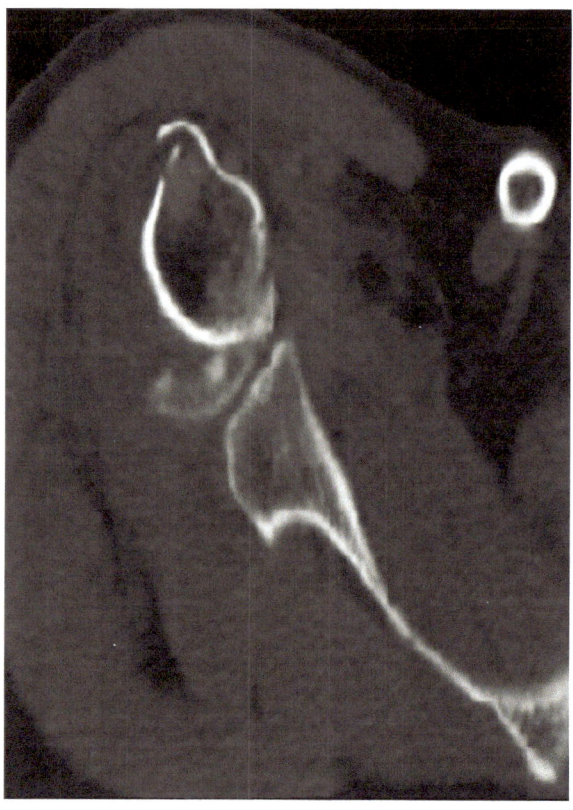

FIGURE 3.16 Axial CT cut exhibiting a coronal fracture line, which was the distal extension of the greater tuberosity fragment

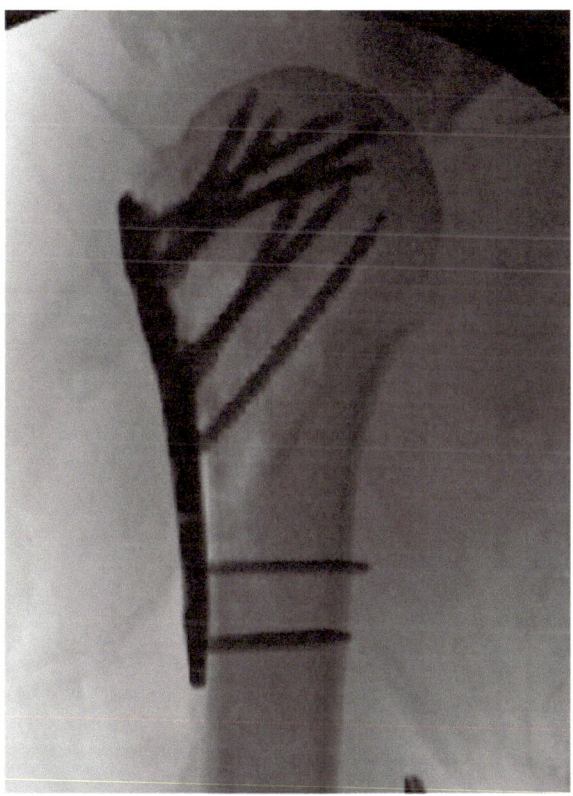

FIGURE 3.17 Again, exposure, suturing of the tuberosities, and proximal fixation followed by a non-locking shaft screw will help achieve a desired reduction

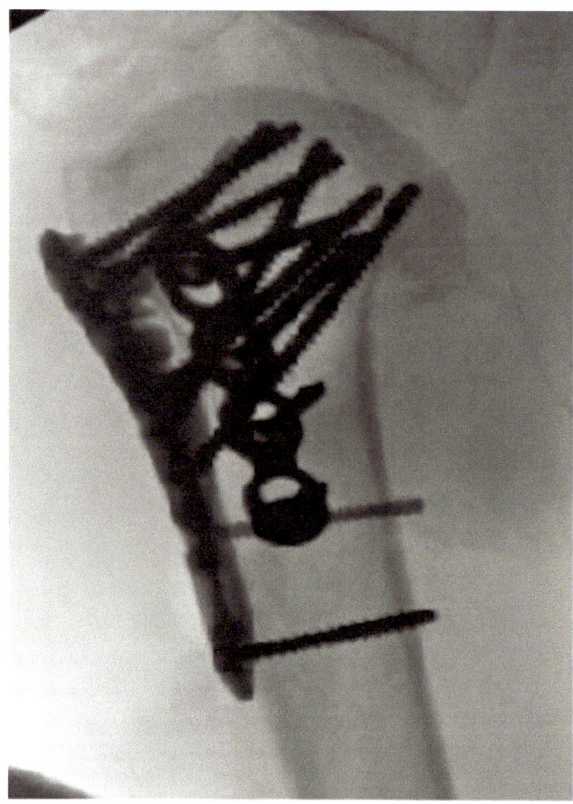

FIGURE 3.18 Intraoperative shoulder range of motion noted gapping of the coronal fracture; thus an additional plate was placed to further strengthen the construct, allowing for early range of motion

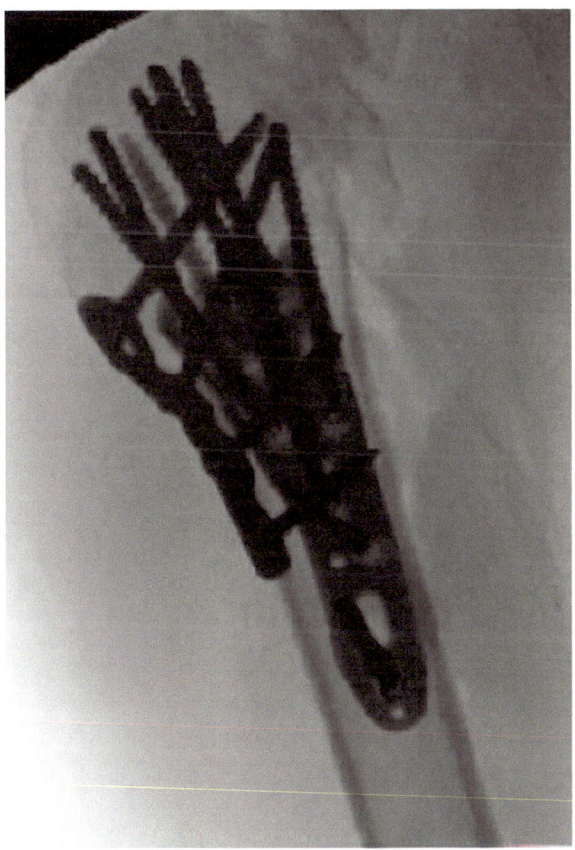

FIGURE 3.19 Dual-plate fixation with a proximal humerus locking plate and 3.5 mm reconstruction plate to buttress the greater tuberosity fragment, with appropriate positioning, and screw lengths on the lateral view

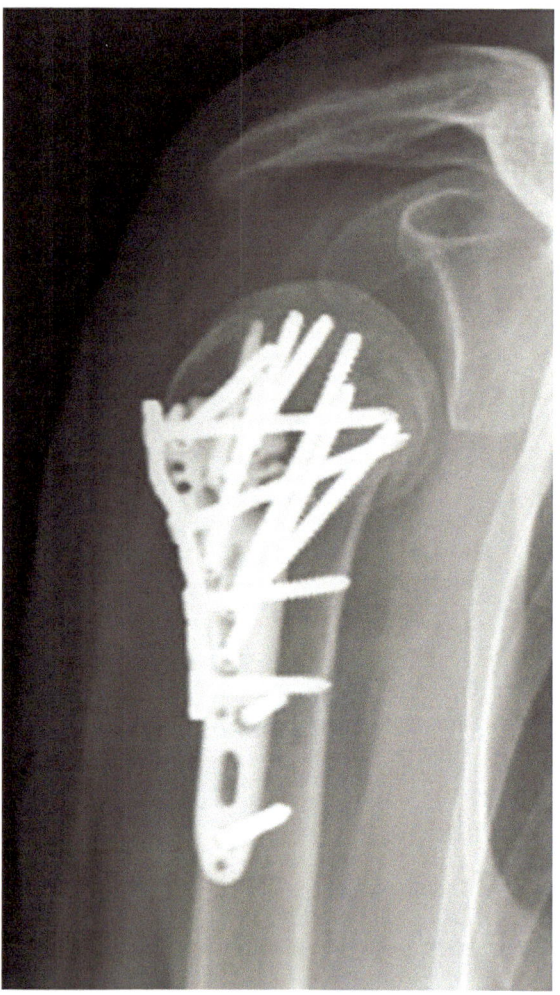

FIGURE 3.20 AP radiograph exhibiting healed fracture. No penetration of the humeral head and appropriate plate placement

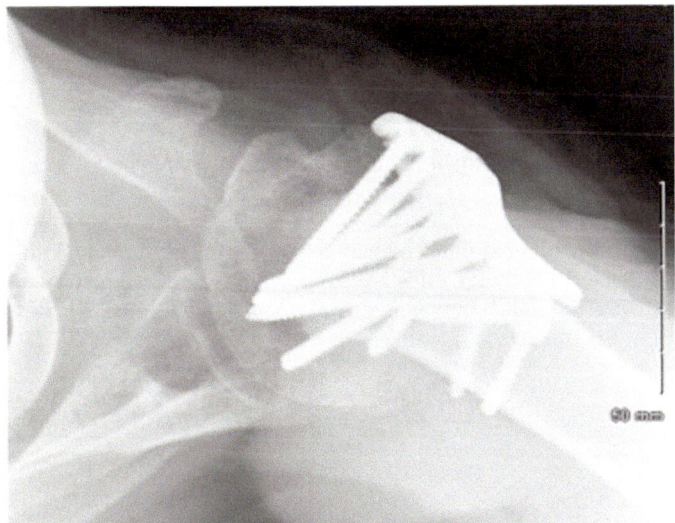

FIGURE 3.21 Axillary radiograph exhibiting healed fracture with appropriate glenohumeral articulation and well-placed hardware

References

1. Streubel PN, Sanchez-Sotelo J, Steinmann SP. Proximal humerus fractures. In: Court-Brown C, Heckman JD, McQueen MM, Ricci WM, Tornetta P, editors. Rockwood and Green's fractures in adults. Philadelphia: Wolters Kluwer Health; 2015. p. 13411425.
2. Schulte LM, Matteini LE, Neviaser RJ. Proximal periarticular locking plates in proximal humerus fractures: functional outcomes. J Shoulder Elb Surg. 2011;20:1234–40.
3. Hasty EK, Jernigan EW, Soo A, Varkey DT, Kamath GV. Trends in surgical management and costs for operative treatment of proximal humerus fractures in the elderly. Healio Orthopedics. 2017;40(4):e641–7.
4. Sudkamp N, et al. Open reduction and internal fixation of proximal humeral fractures with use of the locking proximal humerus plate. J Bone Joint Surg Am. 2009;91:1320–8.

5. Olerud P, Ahrengart L, Ponzer S, Saving J, Tidermark J. Internal fixation versus nonoperative treatment of displaced 3-part proximal humeral fractures in elderly patients: a randomized controlled trial. J Shoulder Elb Surg. 2011;20:747–55.
6. Xie L, Ding F, Zhao Z, Chen Y, Xing D. Operative versus non-operative treatment in complex proximal humeral fractures: a meta-analysis of randomized controlled trials. Springerplus. 2015;4:728.
7. Brunner F, et al. Open reduction and internal fixation of proximal humerus fractures using a proximal humeral locked plate: a prospective multicenter analysis. J Orthop Trauma. 2009;23:163–72.

Chapter 4
Humeral Shaft Fractures

Mai P. Nguyen and Heather A. Vallier

Humeral shaft fractures are defined as fractures from the surgical neck of the proximal humerus to the supracondylar ridge. Approximately 70,000 humeral shaft fractures occur annually and are estimated to be between 3% and 5% of all fractures [1]. These fractures have a bimodal age distribution with low-energy fractures such as falls from standing height in elderly patients and high-energy motor vehicle collisions, contact sports, falls from height, and gunshot injuries in younger patients.

As with all trauma patients, a detailed history and physical examination is an important first step. Advanced Trauma Life Support protocol should be followed and careful attention paid to associated, potentially life-threatening injuries such as

M. P. Nguyen
Department of Orthopaedic Surgery, University of Minnesota, Minneapolis, MN, USA

H. A. Vallier (✉)
Department of Orthopaedic Surgery, Case Western Reserve University, Metro Health System, Cleveland, OH, USA
e-mail: hvallier@metrohealth.org

© Springer Nature Switzerland AG 2020
D. S. Horwitz et al. (eds.), *Tips and Tricks for Problem Fractures, Volume I*,
https://doi.org/10.1007/978-3-030-38274-2_4

scapulothoracic dissociation and pneumothorax. Neurological and vascular evaluation should be performed as injuries are frequent especially after high-energy trauma. The radial nerve is at risk due to its intimate relationship with the shaft in the radial groove. Prophylactic antibiotics should be administered urgently for open fractures, and tetanus immunization should be updated. Patients with ipsilateral humeral and forearm fractures should be closely observed for compartment syndrome. Standard orthogonal imaging should be obtained to view the entire humerus as well as the shoulder and elbow.

Case 1. Non-operative Treatment

The patient is a 50-year-old, right-hand-dominant male who fell from a horse and sustained a right humeral shaft fracture with ipsilateral pneumothorax. He was evaluated in the emergency department and a coaptation splint was placed (Fig. 4.1). Care was taken to position the splint medially into the axilla and laterally over the superior aspect of the shoulder. A cuff and collar fosters positioning of the wrist superior to the elbow, reducing movement in the fracture and aiding in gravity-assisted reduction. He was advised to maintain an upright posture, even while sleeping, to maintain alignment and to reduce pain. One week later the patient was transitioned to a humeral fracture brace. Gentle longitudinal traction is placed on the upper arm while a capable assistant places the brace. Brace shape is customized, especially at the elbow to eliminate skin irritation, and the brace straps are securely fastened. The patient and family were advised to keep the brace on at all times and to tension the straps daily to maintain a snug fit. He was instructed on elbow, forearm, wrist, and hand active and passive motion as well as pendulum exercises for the shoulder. Active-assisted and passive shoulder range of motion exercises were instituted over the next few days. His fracture exhibited abundant callus at 6 weeks (Fig. 4.2), and he was instructed on removing his brace

FIGURE 4.1 Fracture was initially maintained in a coaptation splint

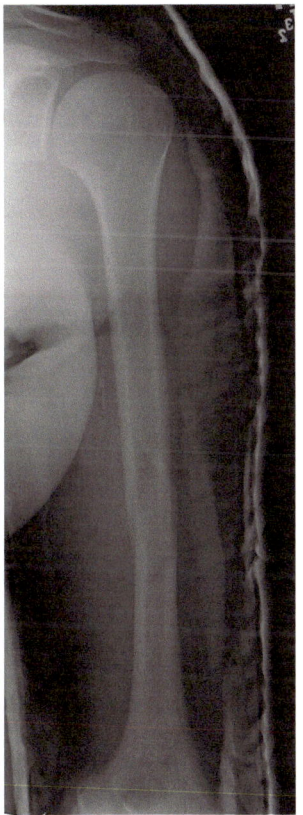

for hygiene only, while continuing brace wear for another 3–4 weeks to protect the maturing bone.

The humerus has a robust, vascularized soft tissue envelope, which facilitates its high union rate, 98% for closed fractures and 94% for open fractures in the Sarmiento series [2]. Most fractures can be treated non-operatively with a coaptation splint followed by fracture brace within 1–2 weeks after injury. Deformities including <20 degrees of angulation in the sagittal plane, <30 degrees of coronal plane or limb shortening <2 to 3 cm are considered acceptable with good function [3] since shoulder and elbow range of motions

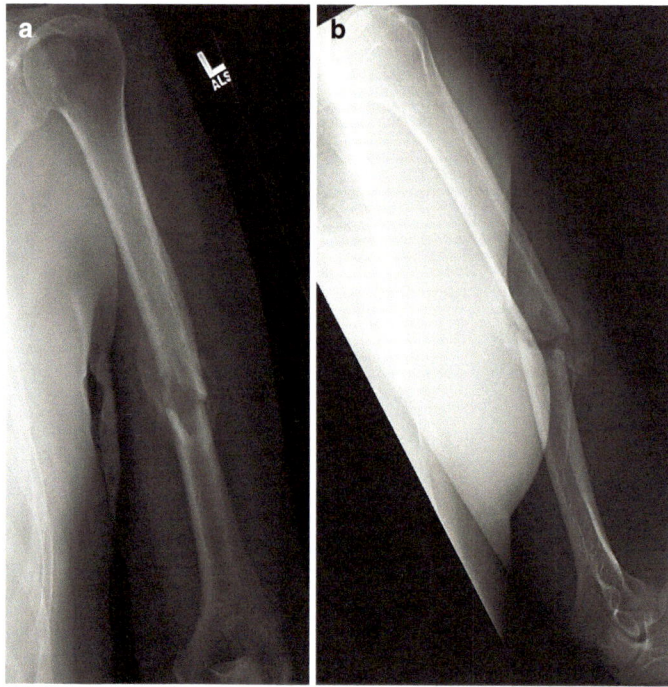

FIGURE 4.2 (**a**, **b**) Bridging callus was visualized at 6 weeks after the injury. The patient reported no pain

accommodate a wide range of radiographic malunion with little or no functional deficit. A minority of patients with isolated humeral shaft fractures benefit from surgical intervention. Indications for surgery include open fractures, associated adjacent articular fractures, ipsilateral forearm fractures, vascular injuries requiring repair, and those with suspected nerve lacerations or loss due to high-energy ballistic injuries or other penetrating trauma. Polytrauma patients with injuries resulting in recumbent positioning are better served with fixation of the humerus because bracing will not be effective unless the patient is upright. Additionally, patients with associated pelvic or lower extremity injuries may be able to utilize an injured humerus shaft for weight bearing if the humerus fracture has been stabilized with a plate or nail. If nonoperatively treated fractures do not exhibit some clinical and radiographic healing within 6 weeks it is advisable to recommend open reduction and internal fixation to achieve expeditious fracture union.

Case 2. Plate Fixation of Comminuted Fracture with Associated Nerve Injuries, Anterolateral Approach

The patient is a 41-year-old-male who sustained multiple gunshot wounds to his dominant right arm resulting in a comminuted humeral shaft fracture with associated radial nerve and musculocutaneous nerve palsies (Fig. 4.3). Vascular status was intact. This case underscores the importance of a detailed physical exam on presentation.

The overall rate of radial nerve palsy associated with humeral shaft fracture is estimated to be 11%, slightly higher for distal third fractures (up to 24%) [4]. Spontaneous recovery is expected in most patients; thus observation is appropriate for the majority of cases. Nerve palsy associated with closed fractures and low-energy ballistic fractures is usually due to neuropraxia, which will recover in most cases, and fracture fixation is not routinely indicated, unless for other reasons. Although associated radial nerve palsy in closed fractures does not warrant nerve exploration, penetrating injuries from sharp object laceration or from high-energy gunshot injuries might cause nerve laceration; thus, exploration may diagnose a nerve discontinuity. These patients are indicated for surgery to reduce and stabilize the fracture and to explore injured nerves.

In this case, the patient was offered surgery for open reduction internal fixation secondary to fracture complexity and to multiple injured nerves. The patient was positioned

54   M. P. Nguyen and H. A. Vallier

FIGURE 4.3
Comminuted
humeral shaft
fracture with
extensive shortening

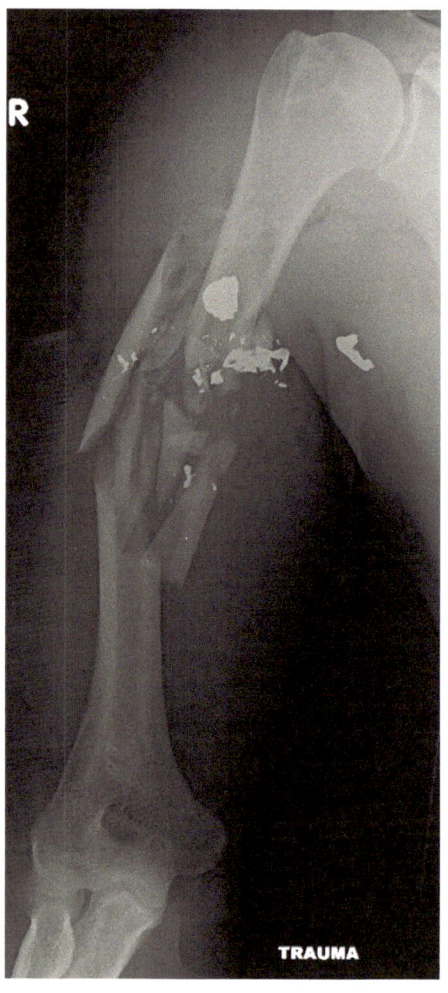

on a table with a radiolucent arm board and the patient was
positioned supine for the anterolateral approach. The endotracheal tube was taped to the opposite side. If planning to
use fluoroscopy or mini C-arm machinery, it may be helpful
to confirm adequate imaging prior to prepping and draping.

Due to the proximal location of fracture sites, tourniquets are not used for most humeral shaft fractures. Hypotension and hemostasis will facilitate visualization of the surgical field.

The deltopectoral approach was made and extended distally into the anterolateral approach to the humerus shaft along the lateral aspect of the biceps and splitting the underlying brachialis. Portions of the deltoid and pectoralis major insertions were elevated from the bone to facilitate plate placement. The radial nerve was identified and assessed from outside the zone of injury between brachialis and brachioradialis distally into the zone of injury and proximally beyond the zone of injury. The musculoskeletal nerve was identified medially and was also noted to be intact throughout its course. A nerve stimulator can be used intraoperatively to help localize the nerves. Once nerves are identified and protected, reduction and fixation of the fracture are undertaken.

This patient had a segmental fracture with several large fragments. Segmental fractures can be challenging to keep reduced and held in place with standard clamps or lag screws alone due to significant torque across the arm. One approach is to sequentially reduce the fractures from proximal to distal or distal to proximal. The reductions can be held temporarily with mini-fragment plates (2.4 mm or 2.7 mm), which can be removed or left in place after final implant placement (Fig. 4.4). Plate choice varies depending on the fracture pattern, bone quality, and size of the patient. Standard large fragment plates are effective in most cases. At least three points of bicortical fixation are recommended on each side of the fracture with a fourth bicortical screw considered for large bridged segments. Screws should be staggered in trajectory to prevent accumulation of a linear stress riser along the far cortex which could result in catastrophic fracture. Comminuted fractures also present a challenge in restoring appropriate alignment. Length may be slightly shortened as needed to enhance bony contact and fracture stability as well

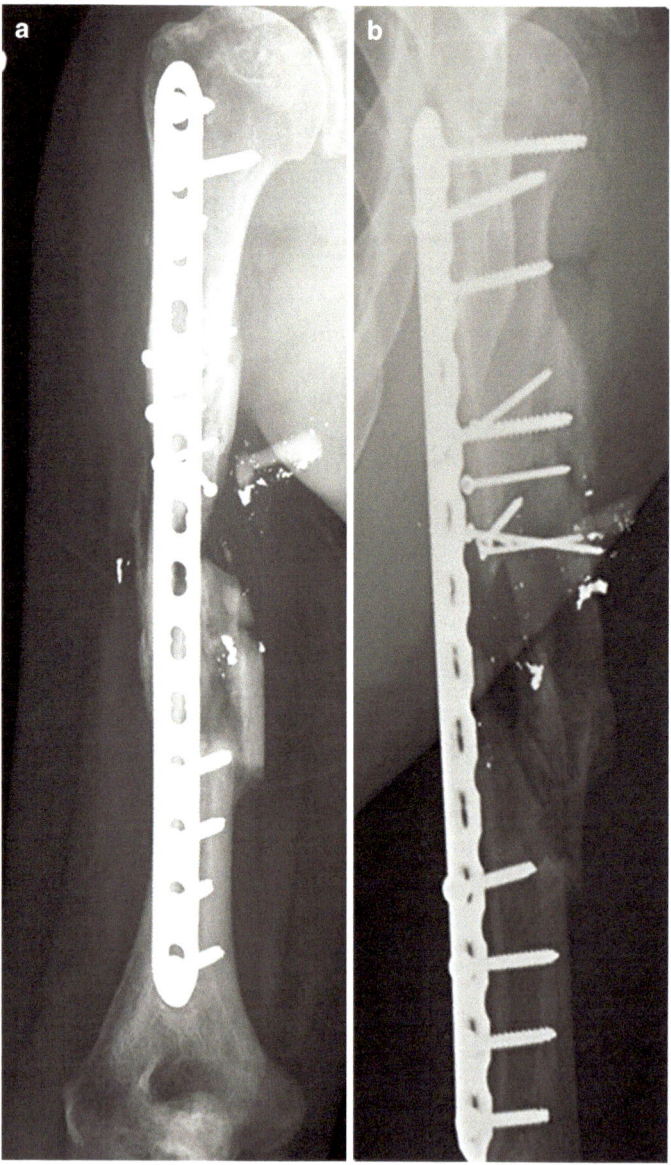

FIGURE 4.4 (**a**, **b**) A large fragment plate was used to bridge the comminuted fracture, including eight cortices of fixation both proximally and distally

as to facilitate healing. Angular alignment may be best assessed intraoperatively with plain radiography. Rotational alignment may also be confusing and may be best assessed with intraoperative plan radiographs as well as clinical and radiographical examination of the contralateral (if unaffected) arm.

In the event of a nerve injury requiring repair, the repair or grafting should occur after fracture fixation to prevent intraoperative re-injury. Postoperatively, the patient was fitted with a wrist and finger extension brace to prevent contracture. He demonstrated some recovery of motor function of both the radial and musculoskeletal nerves after 6 weeks. If no motor improvement is observed, an electromyography may be obtained at 6 weeks and thereafter to monitor nerve recovery.

Case 3. Plate Fixation of a Distal Humeral Shaft Comminuted Fracture with Radial Nerve Injury, Posterior Approach

The patient is a 21-year-old male who sustained a self-inflicted gunshot resulting in distal humeral shaft fracture and associated radial nerve palsy (Fig. 4.5). The radial nerve crosses the posterior aspect of the humerus approximately 20 cm proximal to the medial epicondyle and 14 cm proximal to the lateral epicondyle [5]. Thus, posterior approaches in general provide excellent access to both the radial nerve and the distal humeral shaft. Variations of the posterior approach (paratricepal or triceps-splitting) with radial nerve mobilization allow for exposure of 76–94% of the humerus. In this case, the posterior approach was utilized for exposure of the distal humeral shaft. The patient can be positioned in either the lateral or the prone position. The incision is midline and extends distally lateral to the olecranon fossa. The long head of the triceps is split, and a separate interval adjacent to the lateral aspect of the triceps tendon may be incised to obtain access to the lateral column

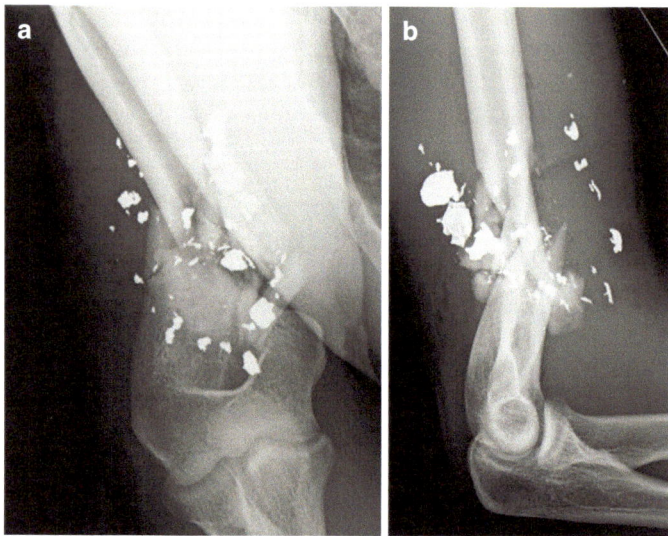

FIGURE 4.5 (**a**, **b**) Comminuted, extra-articular distal humeral shaft fracture

of the distal humerus. The radial nerve is visualized between the long head and the lateral head of triceps. Alternatively, the nerve can be found by following the lateral brachial cutaneous nerve proximally. The nerve is carefully protected intraoperatively, and nerve position with respect to the final plating construct is recorded in the operative record to facilitate nerve identification in the event that secondary procedures are required.

The fracture in this case was quite comminuted. A large fragment plate was used in bridging fashion. Some plates are precontoured to match the distal humeral anatomy, easing implant placement. Screw trajectories must avoid the olecranon fossa and the anterior capitellum. The humeral shaft was slightly shortened to allow for bony contact and to facilitate union (Fig. 4.6). The humerus can tolerate 2–3 cm of shortening without any functional deficit [2, 3].

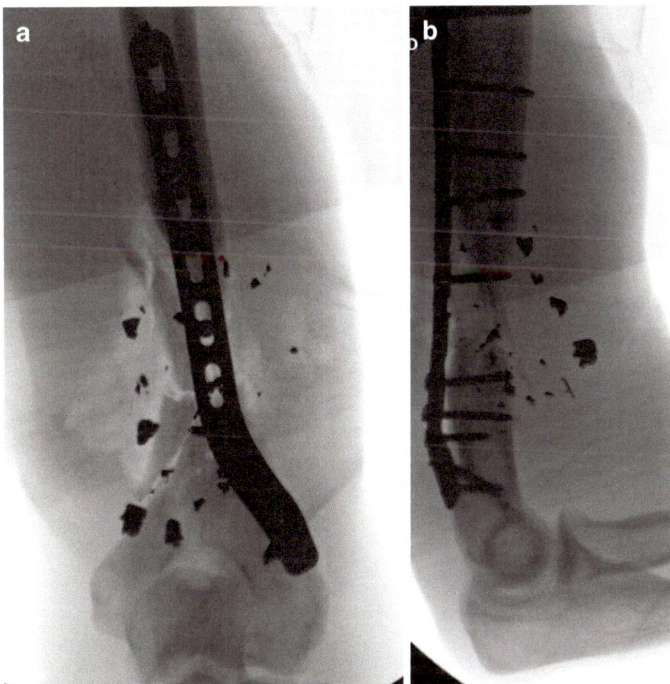

FIGURE 4.6 (**a**, **b**) A large fragment posterolateral plate was placed. The humeral shaft was slightly shortened to provide bony apposition to facilitate union

Cases 4 and 5. Management of Polytrauma Patients

Patients with multiple injuries, including fractures of the pelvis or lower extremities, may benefit from humeral fracture fixation to promote immediate weight bearing on the upper extremities. Case 4 illustrates a 30-year-old male with a pelvic ring injury and a left simple transverse humeral shaft fracture (Fig. 4.7). His pelvic ring fracture limited his weight bearing for 3 months. His transverse humerus fracture was treated with open reduction internal fixation via the anterolateral approach.

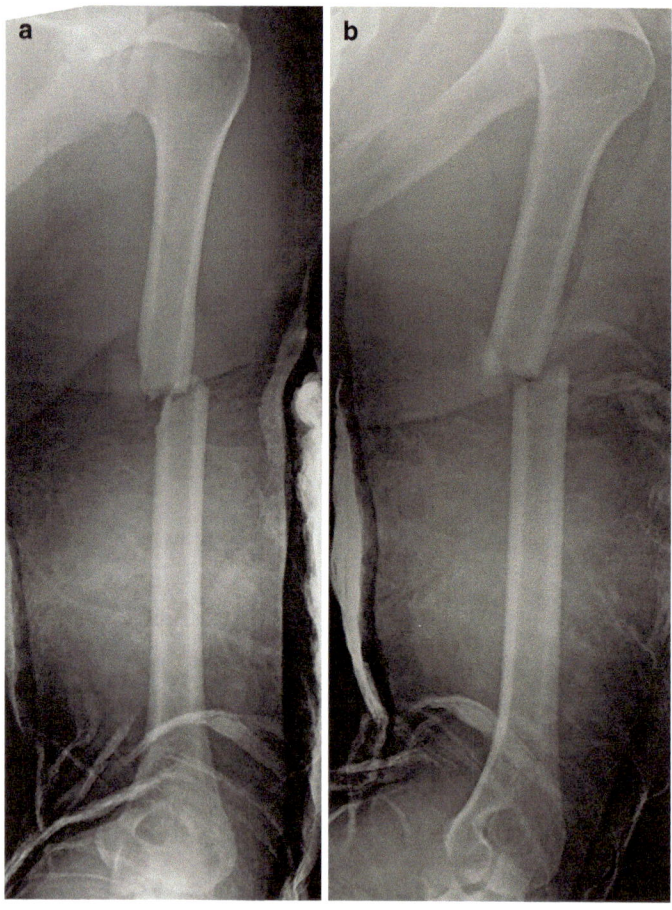

FIGURE 4.7 (**a**, **b**) This polytrauma patient had an unstable pelvic ring injury and a transverse humeral shaft fracture

The fracture was anatomically reduced, compressed and fixed with a narrow 4.5 mm limited contact dynamic compression plate (Fig. 4.8). Pre-bending of the plate and eccentric screw placement promote compression of the fracture. With this rigid construct, the patient was allowed immediate range of motion and weight bearing as tolerated with no splinting.

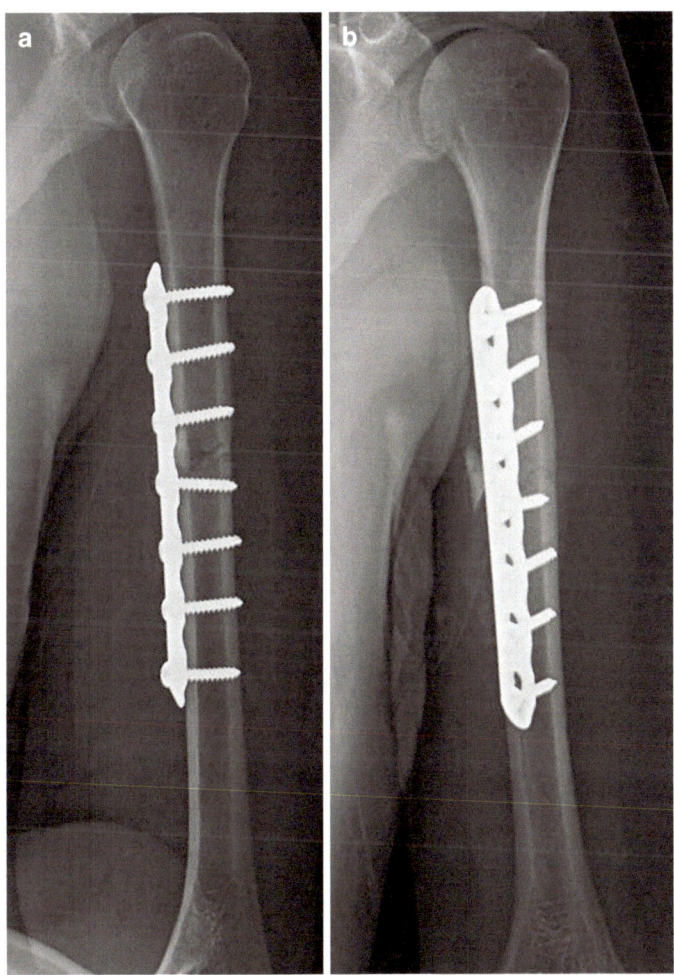

FIGURE 4.8 (**a, b**) Anatomic reduction and compression plate fixation was achieved with this simple transverse fracture

Case 5 depicts a 62-year-old female with left tibial plateau and ankle fractures and right humeral shaft fracture distal to another proximal humeral shaft fracture that she sustained 6 weeks prior (Fig. 4.9). A humeral intramedullary nail was

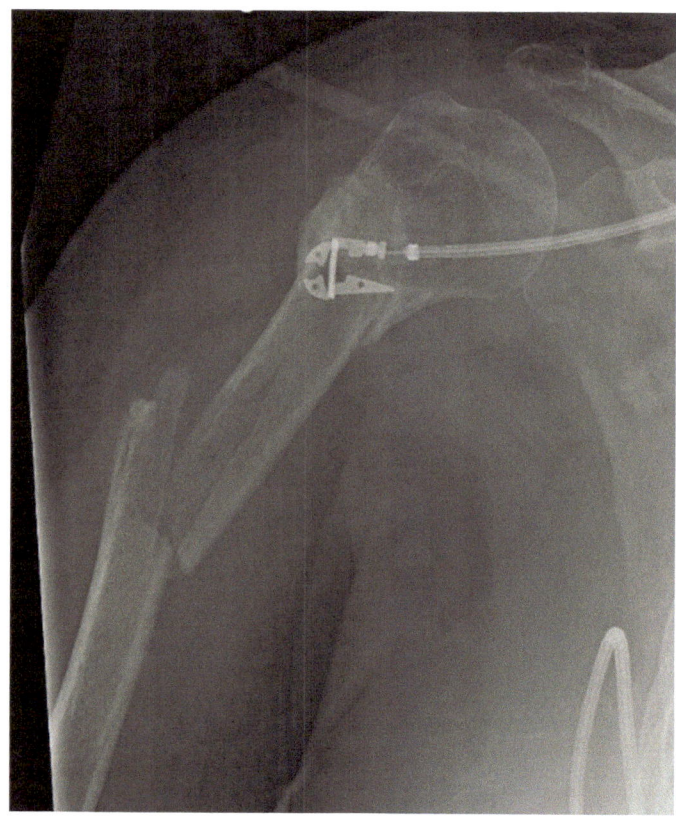

FIGURE 4.9 The patient had multiple extremity fractures including a segmental humeral fracture

used to stabilize both humerus fractures. Intramedullary nails can be placed via a small entry incision (Fig. 4.10). Closed reduction without dissection of the fracture site allowed preservation of periosteal blood supply and minimizes soft tissue trauma [6].

The patient was placed in the supine position at the edge of the bed which allowed for extension of the arm next to the bed. An arm board may be attached to the bed at the level of

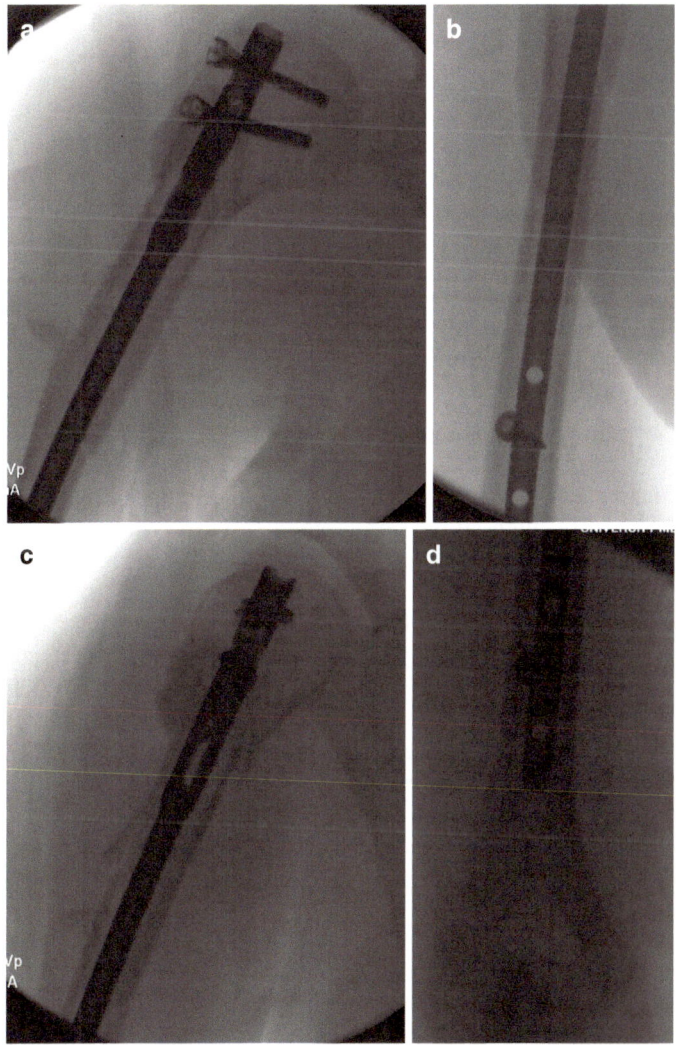

FIGURE 4.10 (a–d) A humeral nail was used to stabilize both humeral fractures

the proximal thigh and rotated toward the patient's forearm to allow to the arm board to support the forearm while keeping the upper arm free. A small bump, such as a folded bath towel, is placed posterior to the scapula to position the shoulder slightly elevated from the table for easier access. A small incision next to the acromion was used and the nail entry was prepared at the rotator cuff interval in order to minimize shoulder pain due to rotator cuff irritation. A guide wire was passed distally across the reduced fracture. Percutaneous Schanz pins or a small incision for clamps or other instruments may facilitate reduction. However, the surgeon must be mindful of local anatomy, especially nerves, which are easily injured. After sequential reaming, a nail of appropriate length and diameter was inserted. Careful attention is needed at the fracture site as the nail passes in order to avoid fracture distraction. Placing of the distal interlocking bolt was performed through an incision large enough to protect adjacent nerves: the radial nerve from lateral to medial screws, and the musculocutaneous nerve from the anterior to posterior screws. Intramedullary locked nails are a load sharing device. The patient was allowed weight bearing as tolerated afterwards.

There have been several studies comparing outcomes of nails versus plates. They demonstrate similar union rates with some showing higher rate of shoulder pain and secondary procedures for nailing [6–8]. With proper patient indication and good techniques, reasonable outcomes can be achieved with intramedullary nailing and with plating for humerus shaft fractures [7].

References

1. Ekholm R, Adami J, Tidermark J, Hansson K, Tornkvist H, Ponzer S. Fractures of the shaft of the humerus. An epidemiological study of 401 fractures. J Bone Joint Surg Br. 2006;88(11):1469–73.
2. Sarmiento A, Zagorski JB, Zych GA, Latta LL, Capps CA. Functional bracing for the treatment of fractures of the humeral diaphysis. J Bone Joint Surg Am. 2000;82(4):478–86.

3. Klenerman L. Fractures of the shaft of the humerus. J Bone Joint Surg Br. 1966;48(1):105–11.

4. Ring D, Chin K, Jupiter JB. Radial nerve palsy associated with high-energy humeral shaft fractures. J Hand Surg Am. 2004;29(1):144–7.

5. Gerwin M, Hotchkiss RN, Weiland AJ. Alternative operative exposures of the posterior aspect of the humeral diaphysis with reference to the radial nerve. J Bone Joint Surg Am. 1996;78(11):1690–5.

6. Park JY, Pandher DS, Chun JY, Md ST. Antegrade humeral nailing through the rotator cuff interval: a new entry portal. J Orthop Trauma. 2008;22(6):419–25.

7. McCormack RG, Brien D, Buckley RE, McKee MD, Powell J, Schemitsch EH. Fixation of fractures of the shaft of the humerus by dynamic compression plate or intramedullary nail. A prospective, randomised trial. J Bone Joint Surg Br. 2000;82(3):336–9.

8. Cheng HR, Lin J. Prospective randomized comparative study of antegrade and retrograde locked nailing for middle humeral shaft fracture. J Trauma. 2008;65(1):94–102.

Chapter 5
Distal Humerus Fractures

Daniela Sanchez and Daniel S. Horwitz

Case Presentation

A 42-year-old man was brought to the emergency department after sustaining a fall from 10 feet while he was working on the roof of his house. He injured the left side of his body and complained of immediate pain and deformity on his left upper extremity. He was initially treated per advanced trauma life support (ATLS) protocols and no life-threatening injuries were documented. He was found to have moderate swelling and deformity at his distal humerus and severe pain with motion. His left upper extremity was warm and well-perfused, sensation intact and had complete motor function of his wrist

D. Sanchez
Musculoskeletal Institute, Geisinger Health System,
Danville, PA, USA

D. S. Horwitz (✉)
Department of Orthopaedic Surgery, Geisinger Health System,
Geisinger Musculoskeletal Institute, Danville, PA, USA
e-mail: dshorwitz@geisinger.edu

© Springer Nature Switzerland AG 2020   67
D. S. Horwitz et al. (eds.), *Tips and Tricks for Problem Fractures, Volume I*,
https://doi.org/10.1007/978-3-030-38274-2_5

and hand. The patient was placed in a left arm splint and x-rays of his left humerus and elbow were obtained (Fig. 5.1). The initial anteroposterior (AP) and lateral radiographs of the elbow showed an intra-articular distal humerus fracture with metaphyseal comminution and varus angulation.

Additional Imaging

Given the complex anatomy of the distal humerus and the intra-articular nature of this fracture pattern, further radiologic imaging is required. Computed tomography (CT) scans help define the intra-articular fracture pattern, identify fractures in the coronal plane and rule out possible associated injuries (i.e., radial head or coronoid fractures) [1]. A good-quality CT scan is essential for preoperative planning, deciding the appropriate surgical approach and implants required for fixation. If available, three-dimensional (3D) reconstruction should be used as it provides a better understanding of the degree of comminution and column involvement and allows for the subtraction of the proximal forearm. Most distal humerus fractures can be fixed through a posterior triceps sparing approach unless a volar shear fracture is seen on the CT scan. In such cases, an olecranon osteotomy is required to expose the anterior surface of the distal humerus and directly reduce the volar fragment [2, 3]. This patient's CT scan is shown in Fig. 5.2.

Preoperative Planning

After reviewing the radiographic studies, the following issues were noted and needed to be considered when deciding the best treatment option for this patient:

1. *Triangle of stability:* The medial and lateral columns were displaced, and there was a separate trochlear fragment with an intra-articular extension. All the components of the triangle of stability were disrupted and needed to be anatomically restored.

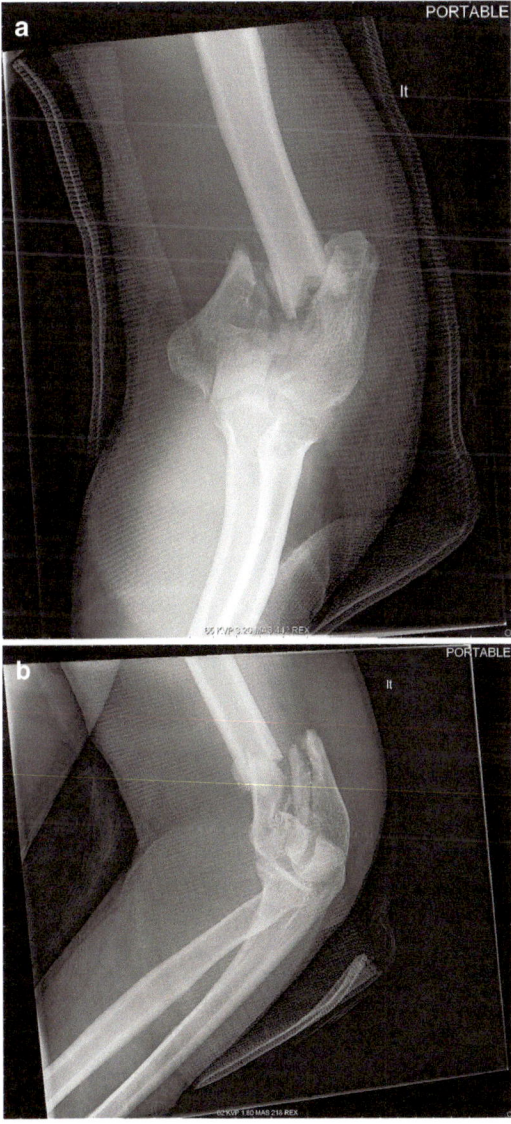

FIGURE 5.1 Initial radiographs of the patient's left elbow show a distal intra-articular humerus fracture. (**a**) AP view showing bicondylar displacement with metaphyseal comminution and a varus angulation of the distal humerus. (**b**) Lateral view shows metaphyseal comminution and a reduced ulnar-humeral joint

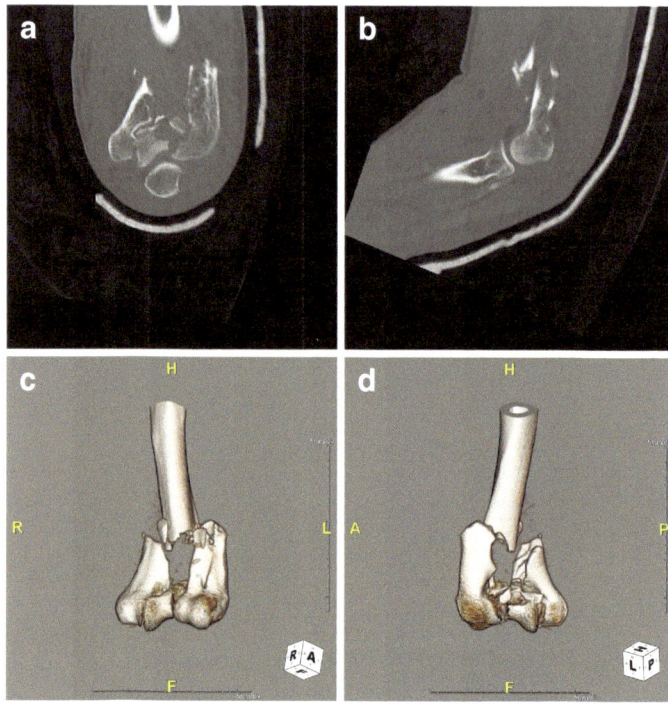

FIGURE 5.2 CT scan of the left distal humerus. (**a**) Coronal cut showing significant metaphyseal comminution with a simple intra-articular extension and a separate trochlear fragment. (**b**) Sagittal cut of the lateral column showing a reduced radio-capitellar joint, no volar shear fracture, metaphyseal comminution and a small distal fragment. (**c**) AP and (**d**) PA 3D-reconstructions of the distal humerus with suppression of the proximal forearm showing a T-type fracture with bicondylar displacement and significant comminution surrounding the olecranon fossa

2. *Comminution:* There was comminution at the metaphyseal-diaphyseal junction and around the olecranon fossa, leaving little bone stock for distal fixation. This degree of comminution also makes inter-fragmentary compression unfeasible due to the risk of over-compression and narrowing the trochlea.

3. *No fractures in the coronal plane:* Without an anterior volar shear fracture, the fracture fragments could be reduced and stabilized through a posterior approach without requiring an olecranon osteotomy.

Open reduction and internal fixation has been the treatment of choice for intra-articular distal humerus fractures. The goal of treatment is to perform an anatomic reduction with fixation stable enough to allow for an early range of motion of the elbow. The medial and lateral columns should be fixed and the triangle of stability must be restored [4].

Patient Positioning

The patient can be placed either in a lateral decubitus or prone position with the arm on a radiolucent support or a padded post allowing elbow flexion beyond 90°. Controlling the patient's airway may be more difficult in a prone position. If a lateral decubitus position is used, the patient needs to be firmly secured to the operating table, often with the use of a bean bag for support of the abdomen, low back, and pelvis. Tourniquet use facilitates visualization at the level of the joint and is routinely used. It is critical to always use foam or silicone dressings at the bony prominences to prevent the formation of pressure ulcers and the peroneal nerve must be well padded on the down leg when in the lateral position.

Intraoperative Imaging

A radiolucent table is generally utilized, and the C-arm can be positioned on the same side or on the opposite side of the table. Positioning the C-arm on the opposite side and coming over the body facilitates obtaining images without disrupting the position of the operating surgeon and assistants. In very unstable fracture patterns or when only provisional fixation has been obtained, the ability to keep everyone in position and minimize the risk of loss of reduction is very appealing.

Implant Choices

Non-anatomic Plates

One-third of tubular plates do not provide enough fixation strength and can easily break; therefore, they should only be used as buttress plates to increase construct stability and not as the single means of fixation. The 3.5-mm pelvic reconstruction plates provide adequate rigidity and are easier to contour, and low-contact dynamic compression plates (LC-DCP) allow the placement of divergent and locked screws providing added fixation with angular stability, but they can be extremely difficult to contour, and distal screw options are limited in comparison to anatomic plates.

Pre-contoured Periarticular Locking Plates

These anatomic plates can be used as a reference for reconstructing the elbow's anatomy and generally offer many options for distal fixation with 2.4-mm and 2.7-mm screws. Lateral, posterolateral, medial, and posteromedial plates are available, and they can be used with either conventional or locked screws. In general, only non-locked screws are required for proximal diaphyseal fixation.

Mini-fragment Plates

These can be used as reduction aids and to fix small fracture fragments to the medial/lateral columns. Often used in combination with anatomic plates, these smaller implants can significantly extend the distal fixation options.

Operative Treatment

The patient was taken to the operating room for open reduction and internal fixation of his fracture, and under general anesthesia he was placed in a lateral decubitus position with a tourniquet on, and his left arm was draped over a padded bolster.

Surgical Approach

The posterior paratricipital approach is triceps sparing and allows the surgeon to work through the lateral and medial windows created by mobilizing the triceps. It also permits the conversion to an olecranon osteotomy (if needed) and lets the patient start immediate active range of motion without concern for olecranon fixation [5].

1. After raising the tourniquet, a long midline skin incision was made over the posterior aspect of the elbow. The incision was curved towards the radial side around the tip of the olecranon.
2. Dissection was carried through the triceps fascia and around the medial and lateral aspects of the triceps to create a medial and lateral window.
3. Medial window: The ulnar nerve was exposed 7–10 cm proximal to the medial condyle and dissected down to the cubital tunnel and 6 cm distally into the forearm. The nerve should generally be released and mobilized anteriorly "as if an ulnar nerve transposition was to be performed" in order to protect it from being injured throughout the procedure. The decision regarding transposition is generally made at the end of the case and is often dependent on the presence of exposed implants in the cubital tunnel. The ulnar nerve is protected with a vessel loop that is tied into a knot without placing a clamp on the end.
4. Lateral window: The radial nerve crosses over the posterior humerus approximately 15 cm above the level of the joint, and if fixation needs to extend above 10–12 cm it is always recommended that the nerve be visualized and protected. The nerve is typically located either by tracing the later cutaneous branch back to the spiral groove or by carefully splitting the triceps 1.5 cm above the tendinous junction and carefully tracing it medially and laterally. The radial nerve, when visualized, should also be carefully protected with a vessel loop.
5. Joint visualization: The posterior fat pad is routinely resected in order to allow visualization as well as to decrease post-operative extension block. Lateral capsular

release is fairly intuitive and simply involves sharp dissection along the posterior and lateral aspect of the condyle with a formal capsulotomy. Medially, the capsular release required for visualization can be less obvious. Release of the posterior bundle of the medial collateral ligament (MCL) is required when treating fractures with intraarticular extension and, in general, we strive to preserve the anterior bundle of the MCL. Although the anterior bundle is usually easily palpated, an easy method of gaining the needed exposure is to "prepare" for an olecranon osteotomy and release the medial capsule until the bare spot of the olecranon is visible. This will, by default, release the posterior MCL bundle, and traction and forearm rotation should provide enough joint visualization. If exposure is not sufficient, an osteotomy can be performed.

Sequence of reduction and fracture fixation Identify the column that has the simpler fracture pattern, reduce it to the humeral shaft and provisionally stabilize it and then provisionally fix the other fracture fragments to this (already restored) column. Once overall anatomic alignment has been achieved sequentially, fix both columns and the trochlea to restore the distal humerus' triangle of stability [4].

Plating constructs Single-plate constructs have proven to be unsuitable for the fixation of bi-columnar distal humerus fractures, and instead two-plate constructs are the gold standard of treatment. Orthogonal plates (usually a posterolateral and a medial plate) allow the placement of screws more distally into the lateral condyle and may facilitate fixation of coronal plane fractures while parallel plate constructs (a medial and a lateral plate) provide sufficient distal fixation for less comminuted fractures. Both constructs have similar biomechanical properties and clinical outcomes and plate position should be based on fracture pattern [6].

Lateral column

In this case, the lateral column, which had a simpler fracture pattern, was reduced and fixed first (Fig. 5.3).

1. Elevation of the triceps and retraction medially to expose and clean the fracture site. The radial nerve was visualized and protected.
2. Under a direct visualization, the lateral epicondyle was reduced to the humeral shaft, and the reduction was maintained using pointed reduction clamps and K-wires.
3. Anatomic reduction was confirmed in the AP and lateral views using fluoroscopic imaging.
4. The reduction was secured using an anatomic posterolateral plate with cortical fixation in the proximal and distal fragments.

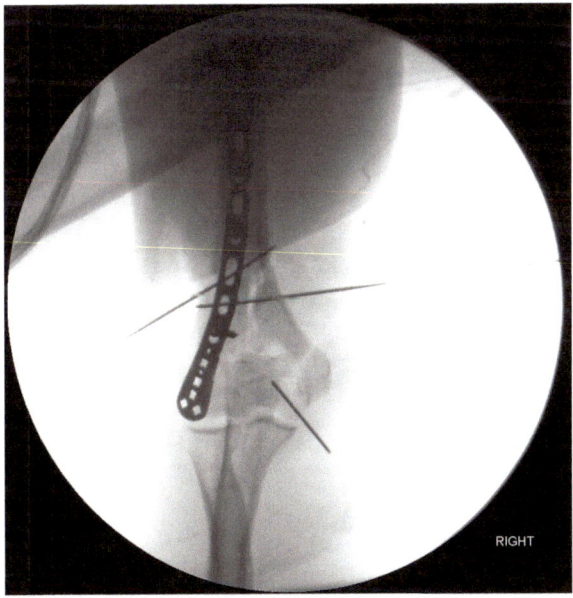

FIGURE 5.3 Fluoroscopic AP view after reduction of lateral and medial columns with K wires in place and a posterolateral column plate in position with proximal fixation only

Medial column

1. Elevation of the triceps and retraction laterally to expose and clean the fracture site. The ulnar nerve was visualized proximally and traced and released into the forearm compartment.
2. Under direct visualization, the fragments of the medial epicondyle were reduced and provisionally fixed, using K-wires, to the humeral shaft and the already restored lateral column.
3. Anatomic reduction was confirmed in the AP and lateral views using fluoroscopic imaging (Fig. 5.3).
4. The most proximal fragment of the medial column was then fixed to the lateral column using an inter-fragmentary compression screw.
5. A medial anatomic plate was placed, provisionally held with K-wires and its adequate positioning confirmed using fluoroscopic imaging.
6. The trochlea was fixed using an inter-fragmentary lateral-to-medial neutralization screw outside the plate.
7. The reduction of the medial column was secured using proximal and distal locking screws and reduction was evaluated in the AP and lateral views using fluoroscopic imaging (Fig. 5.4a). Loss of anatomic reduction was noted, the interfragmentary articular screw and distal medial locked screws were removed, reduction of the trochlea was revised, and after anatomic reduction was confirmed, fixed with a new lateral to medial inter-fragmentary screw (Fig. 5.4b, c).
8. Alternate screw trajectories were used for plate fixation and the final fixation was evaluated using fluoroscopic imaging (Fig. 5.5).

Closure   Wounds were irrigated and closed in a layered fashion. The ulnar nerve was placed back in its anatomic position and an absorbable suture was used to close the soft tissues over the top of the nerve to prevent subluxation

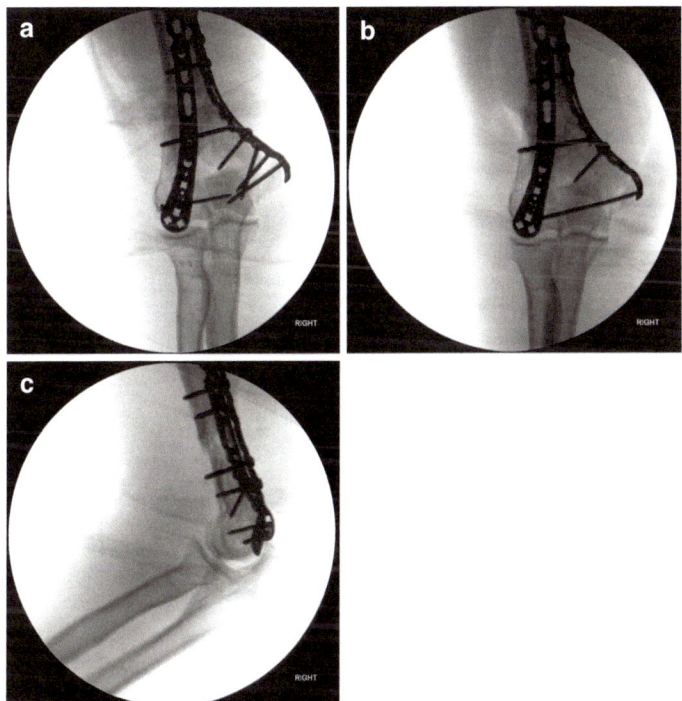

FIGURE 5.4 Fluoroscopic view showing initial reduction and revised reduction. (**a**) Note the gap and step off at the junction of the trochlea and the capitellum. This was deemed to be unacceptable. (**b**) After revision of reduction the medial fixation has been revised, the joint appears anatomically reduced and was now fixed with a lateral to media, longer inter-fragmentary neutralization screw. (**c**) A lateral view confirms alignment in both planes

around the medial epicondyle. Care was taken not to tighten the suture too much around the nerve, and it is imperative that a tonsil clamp can easily slide beneath the suture in order to be sure there is no compression of the nerve itself. The wounds were dressed and the upper extremity immobilized with a posterior splint at 90° of flexion.

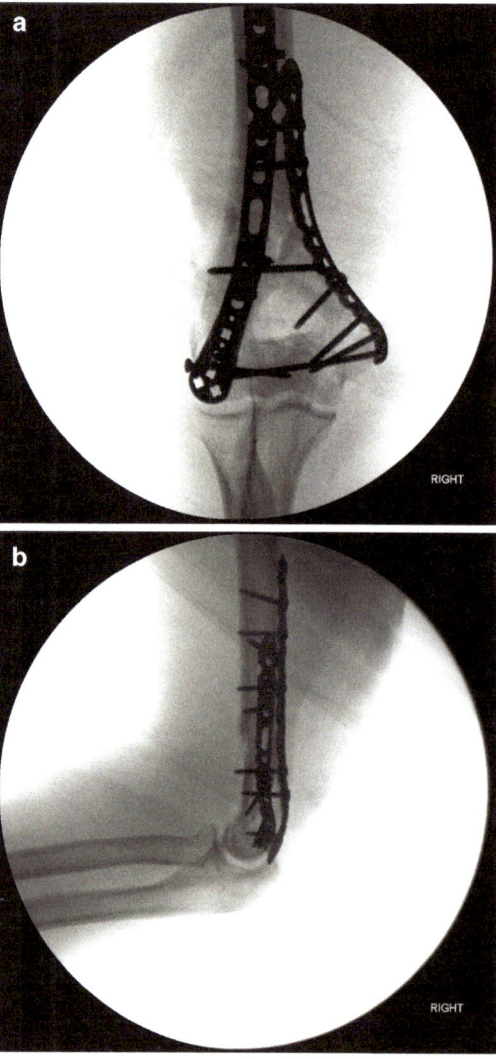

Figure 5.5 AP (**a**) and lateral (**b**) views of the final revised fixation with anatomic alignment confirmed in both planes

Post-operative Protocol and Follow-Up

The patient was kept in a posterior splint for 2 weeks to allow for wound healing. With the goal of early range of motion, the patient was transitioned to a removable posterior molded splint at 2 weeks and allowed to start active and active-assisted flexion and extension of the elbow independently and with physical therapy (PT) supervision. The post-operative course was uneventful, and he progressively gained active range of motion. At 6 weeks, evidence of bone healing were evident (Fig. 5.6), strengthening exercises were initiated, and by 12 weeks the patient had regained near full range of motion with an arc of 5°–140°. At 6 months, the fracture was completely healed (Fig. 5.7), and the patient was allowed to resume all activities as tolerated and discharged from clinic.

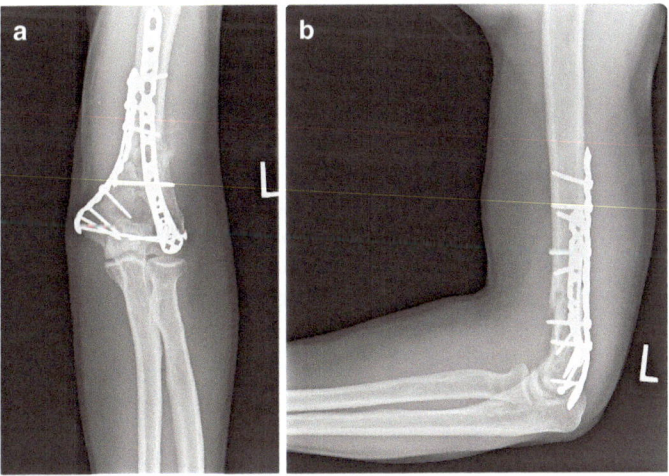

FIGURE 5.6 AP (**a**) and lateral (**b**) views at 6 weeks reveal maintenance of reduction and early callous formation

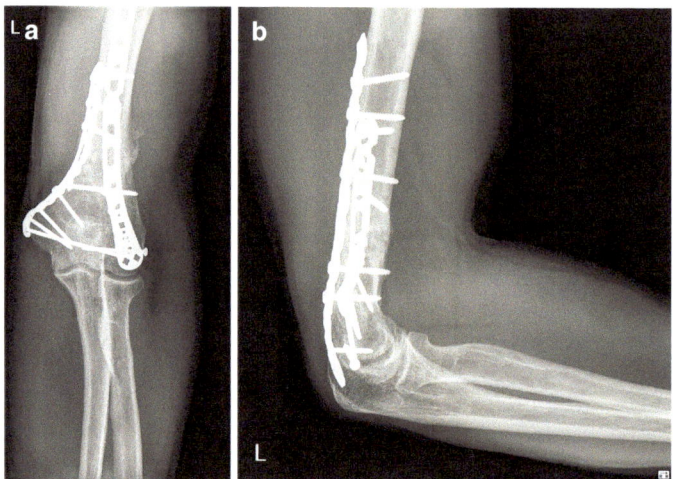

FIGURE 5.7 AP (**a**) and lateral (**b**) views at 6 months show complete healing of all fracture fragments with no loss of alignment

Outcomes

Approximately 80% of patients report good to excellent clinical outcomes after ORIF of distal humerus fractures treated with double-plate constructs [7]. Loss of range of motion may occur, especially terminal extension, and patients should be counseled about this. However, the range of motion after ORIF of type C fractures has reported flexion of 103°–112° degrees and, according to a study published by Morrey et al., most activities of daily living can be performed with 100° of flexion without functional limitations [7, 8].

Summary

The key elements to success in treating this fracture:

1. *Complete understanding of the fracture pattern*

   - Use a CT scan and 3D reconstruction for preoperative planning.

- Most fractures can be fixed through posterior triceps sparing approach unless an anterior volar shear fracture is documented.

2. *Stable patient positioning and fluoroscopic visualization*

- Position the C-arm on the opposite side; this will facilitate obtaining intraoperative images without disrupting flow of surgery.

3. *Adequate joint exposure*

- Resecting the posterior fat pad and releasing the posterior bundle of the MCL.

4. *Adequate exposure and protection of ulnar and radial nerves*

- Release the ulnar nerve as if an ulnar transposition was to be performed.

5. *Planned sequential reduction by column and repetitive visual and fluoroscopic evaluation of this reduction*

- Mini fragment plates can facilitate reduction of smaller fracture fragments.

6. *Readiness to revise fixation*
7. *Initiation of early active range of motion*

References

1. Galano GJ, Ahmad CS, Levine WN. Current treatment strategies for bicolumnar distal humerus fractures. J Am Acad Orthop Surg. 2010;18:20–30.
2. Pollock JW, Faber KJ, Athwal GS. Distal humerus fractures. Orthop Clin North Am. 2017;39(2008):187–200.
3. Zhang C, Zhong B, Cong feng L. Comparing approaches to expose type C fractures of the distal humerus for ORIF in elderly patients: six years clinical experience with both the triceps-sparing approach and olecranon osteotomy. Arch Orthop Trauma Surg. 2014;134(6):803–11.

4. Hessmann MH, Ring DC. Humerus, distal. In: Rüedi T, Buckley R, Moran C, editors. AO principles of fracture management. 2nd ed; 2007. p. 608–25.
5. Alonso-Llames M. Bilaterotricipital approach to the elbow: its application in the osteosynthesis of supracondylar fractures of the humerus in children. Acta Orthop Scand. 1972;43(6):479–90.
6. Steinitz A, Sailer J, Rikli D. Distal humerus fractures: a review of current therapy concepts. Curr Rev Musculoskelet Med [Internet]. 2016:199–206. Available from: https://doi.org/10.1007/s12178-016-9341-z.
7. Reising K, Hauschild O, Strohm PC, Suedkamp NP. Stabilisation of articular fractures of the distal humerus: early experience with a novel perpendicular plate system. Int J Care Inj. 2017;40(2009):611–7.
8. Morrey B, Askew L, Chao E. A biomechanical study of normal functional elbow motion. J Bone Joint Surg Am. 1981;63(6):872–7.

Chapter 6
Olecranon Fractures

Rodrigo Pesantez

Fractures of the olecranon represent approximately 10% of all upper extremity fractures; most of them are the result of a low energy injury, and the most common fracture pattern is a simple displaced fracture (73.5% of these injuries) [1]. Most of them are treated operatively and the goals of treatment are restoration of articular congruity, joint stability and extensor mechanism using a stable fixation that will allow early range of motion.

Preoperative Imaging

Most olecranon fractures are simple and require only an AP and a lateral X-ray of the elbow, but as these fractures become more complex or associated with dislocations of the elbow, additional imaging may be needed, including CT scan

R. Pesantez (✉)
Department of Orthopedic Surgery, Fundación Santa Fe de Bogotá, Bogotá, Cundinamarca, Colombia

© Springer Nature Switzerland AG 2020
D. S. Horwitz et al. (eds.), *Tips and Tricks for Problem Fractures, Volume I*,
https://doi.org/10.1007/978-3-030-38274-2_6

with 3D reconstruction [2]. We prefer to use the Mayo classification [3] as it assesses displacement, comminution and subluxation or dislocation of the elbow.

Planning

Based on the fracture pattern, most transverse and simple fractures are treated in our practice using a tension band wiring technique. More complex fracture patterns or those associated with a dislocation of the elbow are often preferentially treated with dorsal plating.

- Instruments:
    - Senn and small pointed Hohmann retractors
    - Small periosteal elevator
    - Pointed reduction clamps
    - Kirschner wire bender and cutter
- Implants
    - Kirschner wires 1.6 mm/1.2 mm
    - 18 gauge cerclage wire
    - One third tubular plates/periarticular anatomical olecranon plates
    - Mini fragment plates and screws (Hand or Foot set)
    - 3.5 mm pelvic screws

Patient Positioning

For most olecranon fractures a lateral decubitus position with the arm over a radiolucent support or a bolster, making sure the elbow can be flexed and confirming the ability to obtain good imaging with the image intensifier before prepping and draping (Fig. 6.1a–c). Some of these fractures may be treated with the patient supine with the injured arm over the chest, especially simple fracture patterns or a trauma patient who cannot be positioned on their side (Fig. 6.1d).

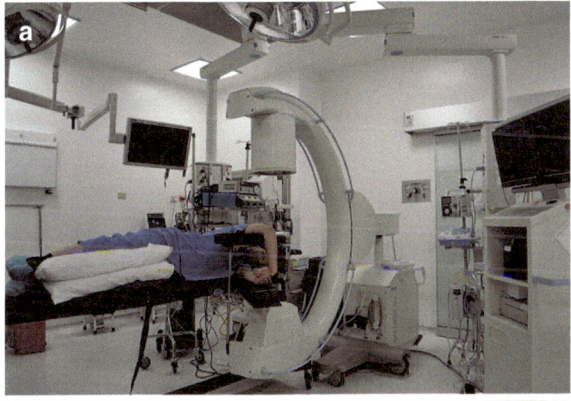

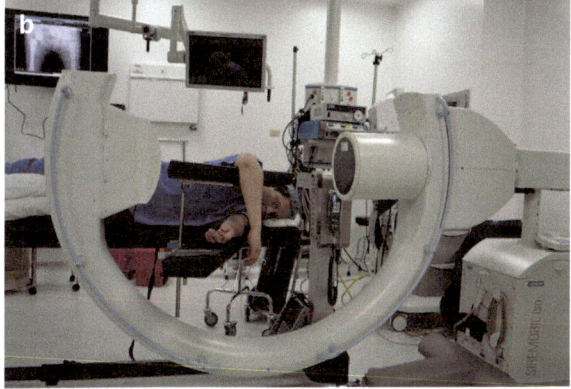

FIGURE 6.1 Patient positioning. (**a–c**) shows the patient position in the lateral decubitus position as well as the position of the C-arm. (**d**) Shows patient supine with the injured arm over the chest

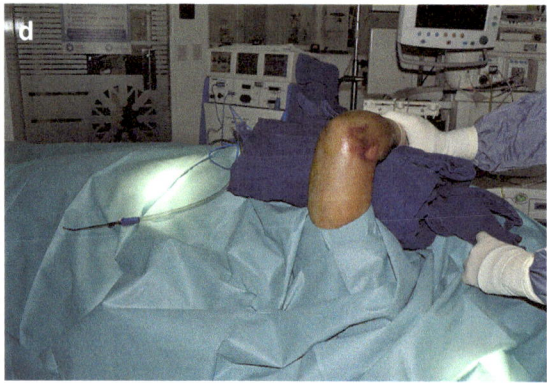

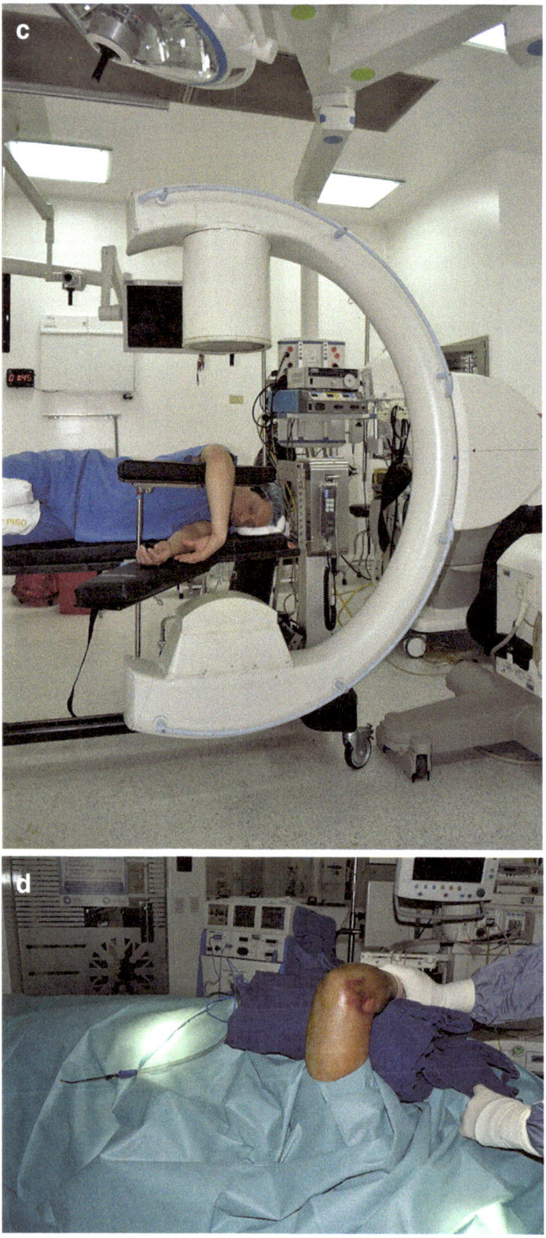

FIGURE 6.1 (continued)

Surgical Approach

Skin Incision

Dorsal longitudinal skin incision, avoid the olecranon process toward the radial side and return to midline. Expose the proximal ulna using full thickness skin flaps, and if you need to expose the ulnar side, identify and protect the ulnar nerve.

Simple Fracture Pattern (Transverse or Short Oblique)

A 27-year-old woman fell off a bike while going to work, and she sustained an isolated right elbow injury. AP and lateral X-rays of her elbow showed a simple displaced transverse olecranon fracture (Fig. 6.2).

In this type of fracture pattern our preferred method of fixation is tension band wiring using Kirschner wires and 18 gauge wire.

Once the fracture edges are exposed 2 mm on either side using a small periosteal elevator, the fracture hematoma is

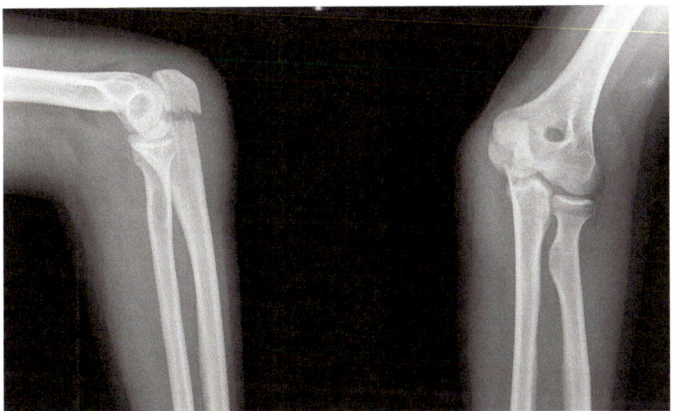

FIGURE 6.2 Simple displaced transverse fracture

cleaned; fracture reduction is performed using a large pointed reduction clamp on each side of the fracture, often making a drill hole using a 2.0 mm drill bit in the dorsal aspect of the ulna to facilitate clamp application (Fig. 6.3).

Expose the articular surface through a small incision in the capsule on the lateral side to assess fracture reduction, and once it is confirmed drill two 1.2–1.6 mm Kirschner wires across the fracture starting dorsal proximal and direct them distal volar in order to anchor the wires distal to the coronoid process and avoid pin migration. Once past the distal cortex back up the wires 5–10 mm in order to allow room for later impaction.

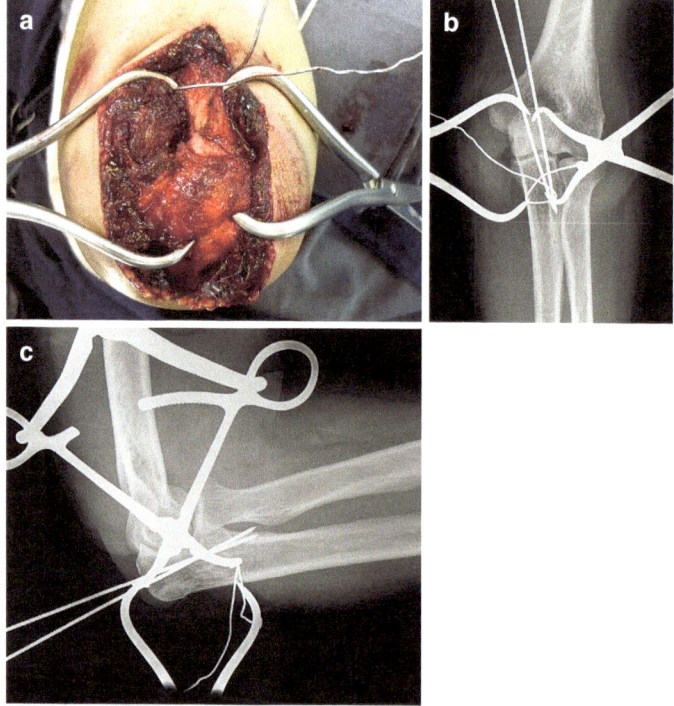

FIGURE 6.3 Fracture reduction using pointed reduction clamps and wire in distal fragment. (**a**) Clinical imaging. (**b**, **c**) X-rays showing fracture reduction and fixation using K-wires

Make a 2 mm drill hole in the apex of the ulna diaphysis distal to the fracture and pass an 18-gauge wire; make a figure of eight and pass it around the Kirschner wires and underneath the triceps tendon using a large-bore needle. Tension each wire medially and laterally twisting them with a wire holder; make the knots less prominent and bend it into the soft tissues.

Bend the Kirschner wires 180 degrees; cut them and impact them into the proximal olecranon using an impactor (Fig. 6.4).

Complex Fracture Patterns and Fracture Dislocations

A 20-year-old male sustained isolated left elbow trauma in a motor vehicle accident. AP and lateral X-rays showed a complex olecranon fracture (Fig. 6.5a). As this is a complex fracture pattern a CT scan (Fig. 6.5b–d) with 3D (Fig. 6.5e–g) reconstruction of his elbow was taken and it shows a comminuted intraarticular and metaphyseal fracture.

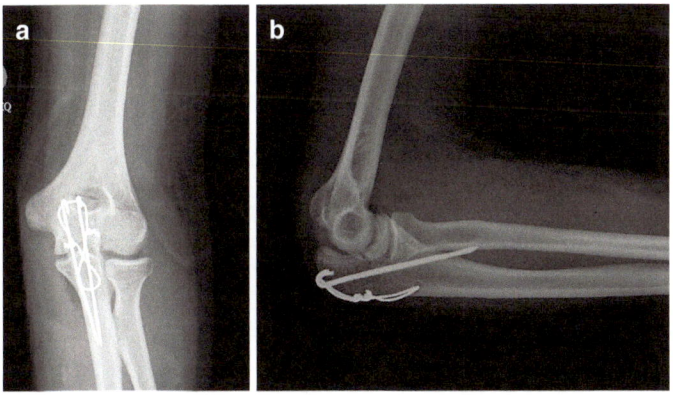

FIGURE 6.4 Final x rays with a tension band wiring of a simple transverse olecranon fractures

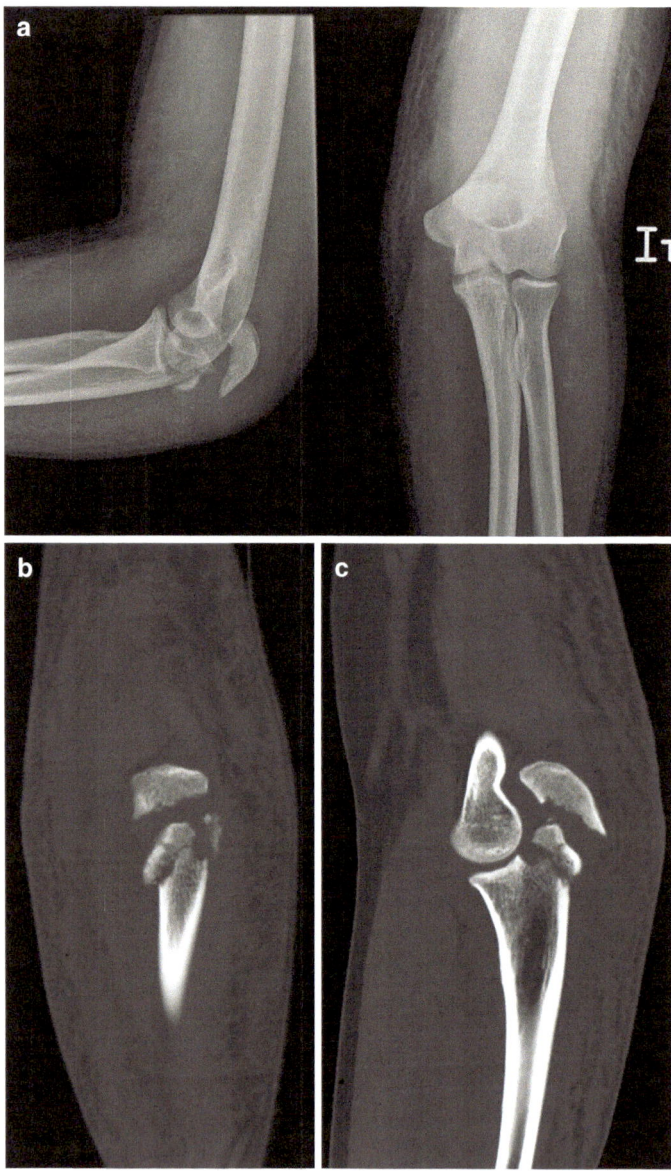

FIGURE 6.5 (a) AP and lateral X-rays of a complex olecranon fracture. (b) Coronal. (c) sagittal. (d) Axial cuts showing metaphyseal and articular comminution. (e–g) 3D reconstruction of the injury

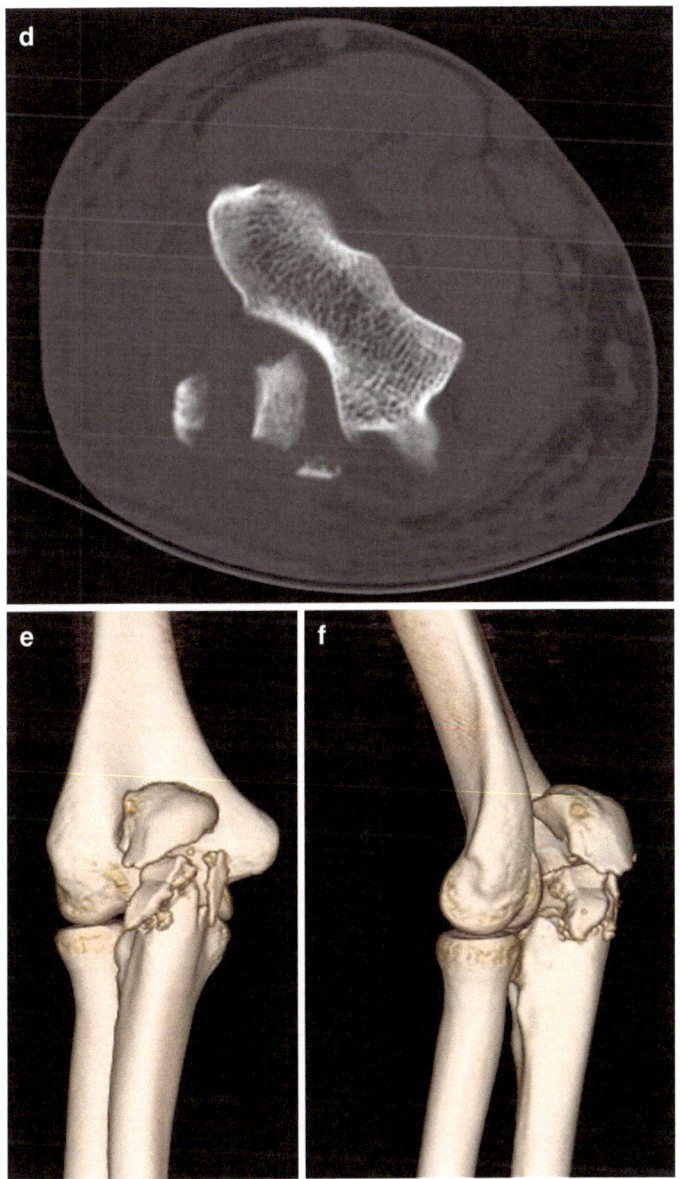

FIGURE 6.5 (continued)

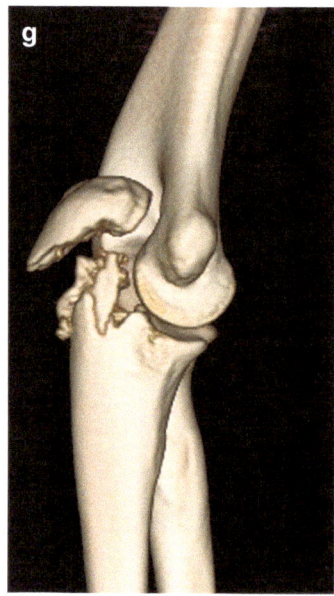

FIGURE 6.5 (continued)

For this type of injury we prefer plate fixation, in young patients with good bone we use one third tubular plates for fixation and for older patients or fracture dislocations we prefer anatomical precontoured plates with locking screw options. In complex intraarticular fractures or with comminution in the metaphysis, we use mini fragment plates and screws as reduction aids and as an adjunct to definitive fixation.

Initial Fixation Through the Fracture

Once the fracture edges are exposed 2 mm on all sides using a small periosteal elevator and the fracture hematoma is cleaned, we assess the articular surface by turning the proximal fragment 90 degrees, exposing the articular surface on both sides, reducing it anatomically, and stabilizing small fragments using temporary Kirschner wires or mini fragment screws buried in the fragments.

Provisional reduction tools (maintaining reduction): Once the main articular fragments have been reduced, assess metaphyseal comminution, and if necessary treat this comminution using mini fragment plates on the medial or lateral side of the proximal ulna. Maintain the reduction using pointed reduction clamps and temporary 1.2/1.6 mm Kirschner wires outside the planned plate position (Fig. 6.6).

Assessing Reduction

The articular surface reduction is assessed once the reduction and fixation of intraarticular fragments is done, and the fracture is reduced and is maintained with temporary fixation. The use of an incision in the lateral or ulnar aspect of the capsule and direct visualization of the joint are an option; otherwise use of the image intensifier in the AP and lateral-planes can confirm articular reduction.

Plate Contouring

The use of aluminum templates as a guide to simply bend a one third tubular plate 90 degrees between the second or third hole, depending on the size of the patient, allows for accurate contouring of these simple plates. Be sure you have at least two or three screws in the proximal fragment, and if the plate is bent in this way one of the screws can go into the tip of the olecranon, another long intramedullary screw can be placed (from the pelvis set), and, if needed, a third oblique screw directed toward the anterior ulnar cortex in the distal fragment can be placed.

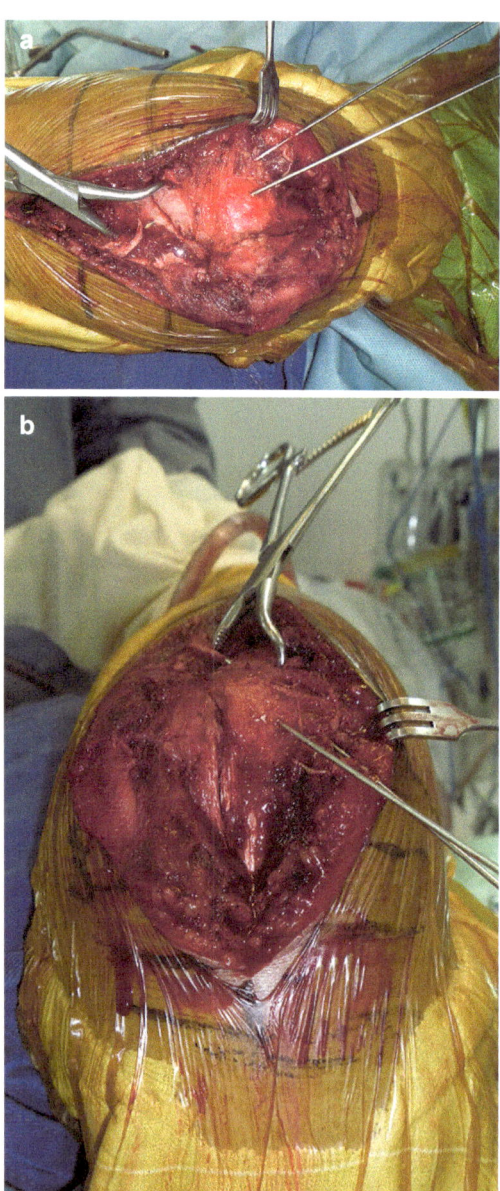

Figure 6.6 Fracture reduction using pointed reduction clamps and temporary Kirschner wire fixation

Triceps Incision

In order to allow the plate to have direct contact with the bone of the proximal ulna, the triceps should be incised and elevated partially medially and laterally (Fig. 6.7).

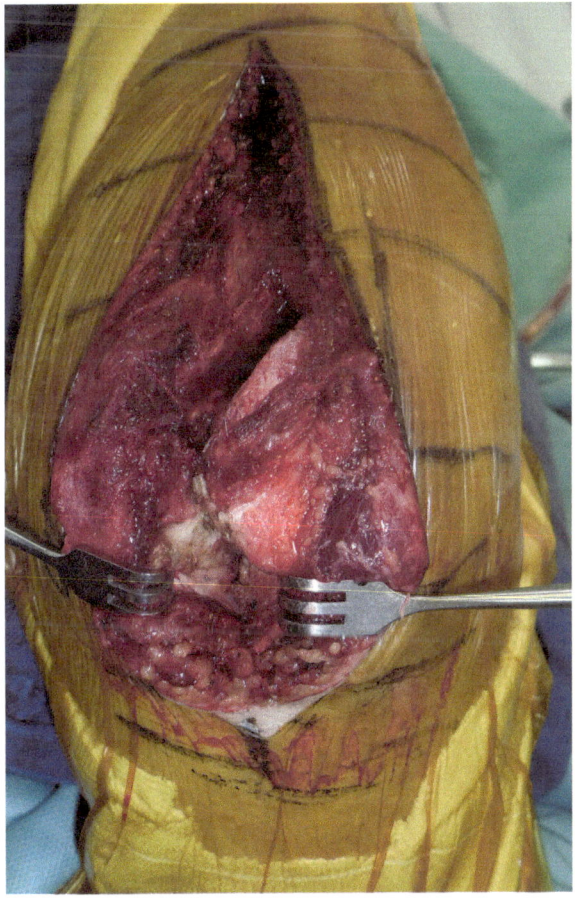

FIGURE 6.7 Triceps incision to expose the tip of the olecranon to apply the contoured plate

Plate Seating

Once the plate is contoured, fix it to the proximal fragment. The first screw placed is the screw from proximal to the bend of the plate toward the tip of the olecranon; this screw will seat the plate to the olecranon (Fig. 6.8). Using the plate-olecranon tip construct, reduce it to the distal fragment and hold the reduction using a Verbrugge or a pointed reduction clamp, holding the plate to the ulnar shaft. Restore the articular congruity of the greater sigmoid notch; review articular and metaphyseal reduction and alignment as well as elbow range of motion and stability. Once all this is done, fix the plate distally with three 3.5 mm cortical screws and finish with two more screws in the proximal fragment: a long intramedullary screw from the tip to the ulnar diaphysis and another from the top-most proximal hole toward the dorsal ulnar cortex. The long intramedullary screw can be also be directed toward the anteromedial ulnar cortex (anterior to the coronoid process to avoid the proximal radio ulnar joint). Mini plates are used for reduction/fixation of smaller fragments: in cases of metaphyseal comminution, additional mini plates from the hand or foot set can be used as temporary or definitive fixation (Fig. 6.9).

Suturing the Triceps

Once the fixation is finished and intraoperative imaging shows an anatomic reduction and restoration of stability, the triceps tendon is sutured over the plate using absorbable sutures.

Wound Closure and Dressing

The wound is closed in a traditional manner, and a soft tissue dressing is put over the wound.

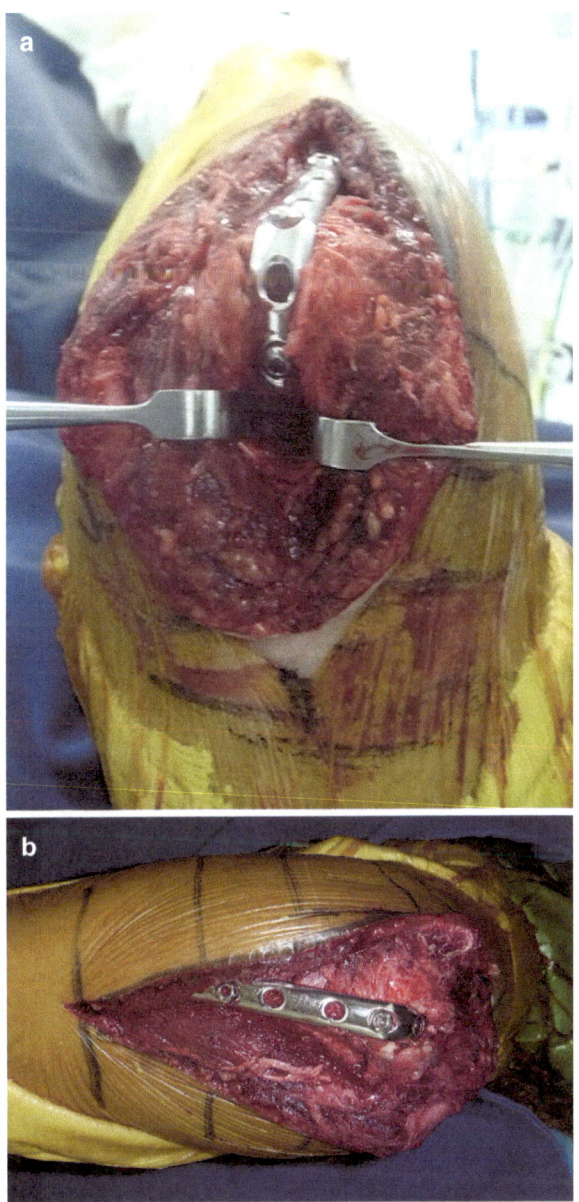

FIGURE 6.8 Plate position in the olecranon tip and the ulnar diaphysis

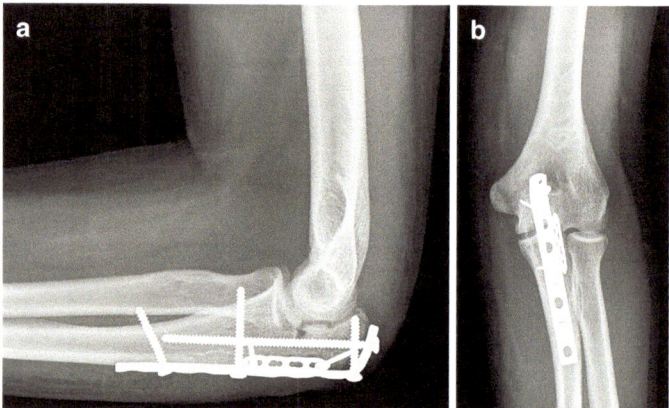

FIGURE 6.9 Final X-rays showing the use of a small fragment 2-mm plate with two screws to address lateral metaphyseal comminution

Postoperative Care

Immediate range of motion is encouraged from day one; weight lifting is restricted for 8–12 weeks. X-rays are taken at 6 weeks, 12 weeks, and 1 year after the injury. Hardware removal is done if requested by the patient once the fracture has healed (Fig. 6.10).

Outcomes

DelSole compared the outcome of 48 olecranon fractures, 23 treated by tension band wiring and 25 with olecranon plating using a hook plate. The fractures were similar in demographics and Mayo classification, and they found that both techniques have similar excellent outcomes, but the plating group had longer time to union and worse terminal extension than the tension band wiring group [4]. In a recent meta-analysis by Ren, a review of 13 studies (1 RCT and 12 observational) comparing tension band wiring with plate fixation was done. They conclude that there are no significant differences in DASH, ROM, operative time, and blood loss between these two techniques, but plate fixation has less complications [5].

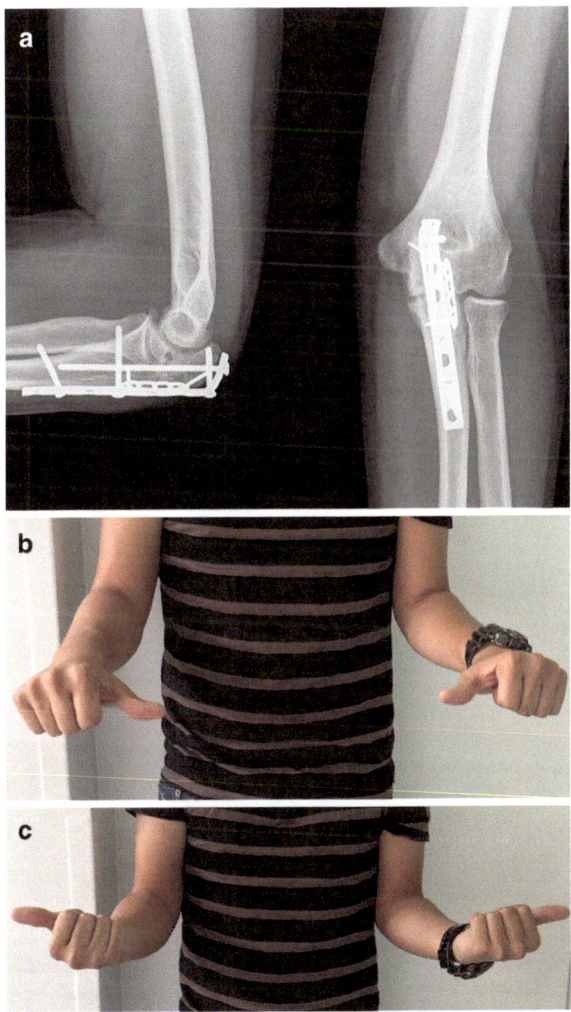

FIGURE 6.10 One year follow-up of the complex olecranon fracture. (**a**) X-rays showing anatomic reduction. (**b–f**) Clinical picture of elbow range of motion. (**g–h**) After removal of the one third tubular plate

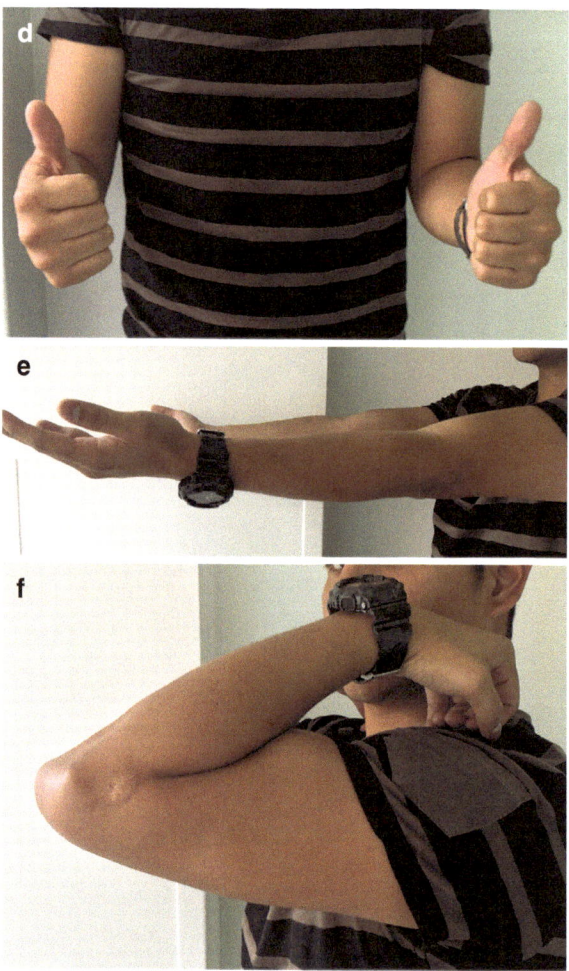

FIGURE 6.10 (continued)

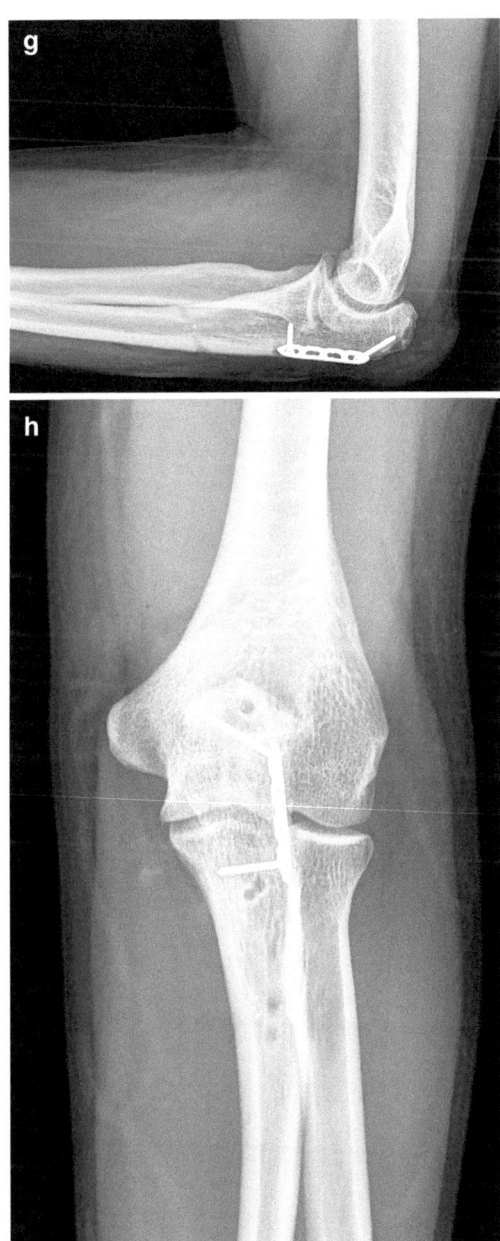

Figure 6.10 (continued)

References

1. Duckworth AD, Clement ND, Aitken SA, et al. The epidemiology of fractures of the proximal ulna. Injury. 2012;43:343–6.
2. Lubberts B, Mellema JJ, Janssen SJ, Ring D. Fracture line distribution of olecranon fractures. Arch Orthop Trauma Surg. 2017;137:37–42.
3. Morrey BF. Current concepts in the treatment of fractures of the radial head, the olecranon and the coronoid. J Bone Joint Surg Am. 1995;77A:316–27.
4. DelSole EM, Pean CA, Tejwani NC, Egol KA. Outcome after olecranon fracture repair: does construct type matter? Eur J Orthop Surg Traumatol. 2016;26(2):153–9.
5. Ren YM, Qiao HY, Wei ZJ, Lin W, Fan BY, Liu J, Li A, Kang Y, Liu S, Hao Y, Zhou XH, Feng SQ. Efficacy and safety of tension band wiring versus plate fixation in olecranon fractures: a systematic review and meta-analysis. J Orthop Surg Res. 2016;11(1):137.

Chapter 7
Radial Head Fractures

Benjamin Richards Wagner and C. Liam Dwyer

Radial head fractures are the most common fractures about the elbow [1]. They typically occur in individuals at a mean age of 48 years and have a slightly higher incidence in women compared to men [2]. While low-energy mechanisms of injury can lead to isolated radial head fractures, higher-energy mechanisms often have associated injuries. The radial head plays a significant role in elbow stability, which is important to consider when treating these fractures. In general, truly nondisplaced fractures may be treated nonoperatively. However, fractures with significant displacement or associated injuries should be treated surgically. Surgical interventions include open reduction internal fixation (ORIF) and radial head replacement. Fragment excision and radial head resection are alternative, although less common, options. This chapter will discuss the presentation and workup of a radial head fracture and then highlight the surgical technique for ORIF and replacement.

_____

B. R. Wagner · C. L. Dwyer (✉)
Department of Orthopaedics, Geisinger Medical Center,
Danville, PA, USA
e-mail: ldwyer@geisinger.edu

© Springer Nature Switzerland AG 2020
D. S. Horwitz et al. (eds.), *Tips and Tricks for Problem
Fractures, Volume I*,
https://doi.org/10.1007/978-3-030-38274-2_7

The radial head articulates with the capitellum and the proximal ulna. Both articular surfaces are important when considering treatment. Biomechanically, axial load transfer through the elbow occurs with roughly 60% through the radiocapitellar joint and 40% through the ulnohumeral joint [3]. The radial head plays an important role as a secondary stabilizer to valgus, posterolateral rotatory instability, and axial stability at the elbow. While other soft tissue and bony structures may act as primary stabilizers to these stresses, they are often concomitantly injured and the importance of the radial head becomes magnified. Important lateral ligamentous structures include the annular ligament, the radial collateral ligament and the lateral ulnar collateral ligament (LUCL).

Fractures of the radial head typically result from a fall onto an outstretched hand with the forearm in pronation and an axial load across the elbow. Associated injuries occur frequently and include medial and lateral collateral ligament injuries, capitellum fractures or chondral injuries, interosseous membrane (IOM) injuries as part of an Essex-Lopresti lesion, coronoid fractures, and olecranon fractures. Fractures of the coronoid and olecranon should raise suspicion for a terrible triad injury (combination of coronoid fractures, radial head fracture, and LCL disruption) and transolecranon fracture dislocations, respectively. Associated injuries should be identified if present and treated appropriately.

Patients often complain of lateral elbow pain and limited range of motion, especially with pronation and supination. Examination should include palpation of the lateral epicondyle, radial head, medial epicondyle, coronoid, olecranon, interosseous membrane, and wrist. Range of motion should assess the amount of elbow flexion, extension, pronation, and supination. A mechanical block to motion should be detected on physical exam. In order to distinguish between a block to motion and limitation secondary to pain, the physician may reevaluate 1 week after injury or aspirate the elbow hemarthrosis and inject local anesthetic prior to examining range of motion. Extremes of motion can be expected to be decreased in the acute setting secondary to soft tissue swelling and may not represent true structural blocks to motion. Attention should also be placed on the distal radial ulnar joint (DRUJ); stability should be tested and compared to the contralateral extremity. Lastly, a thorough neurovascular examination should be performed on all patients.

Imaging of radial head fractures should include anterior-posterior (AP), lateral, and oblique radiographs of the elbow (Fig. 7.1). Swelling and inability to fully extend the elbow may make it difficult to obtain a useful AP image. In this scenario, two separate images, an AP of the distal humerus and an AP of the forearm, may be more useful. An additional radiocapitellar view can help to visualize the radial head in profile. The elbow is positioned for a lateral image and the beam is angled 45 degrees cephalad [4]. The sail sign, anterior or posterior fat pad sign secondary to hemarthrosis, may be present and indicates an occult fracture. In addition, any patient with wrist pain should undergo bilateral PA radiographs at the wrist. Advanced imaging with a CT scan may be obtained in comminuted fractures to assess fragment size and fracture pattern. MRI to evaluate soft tissue injuries has not been shown to significantly change patient treatment [5].

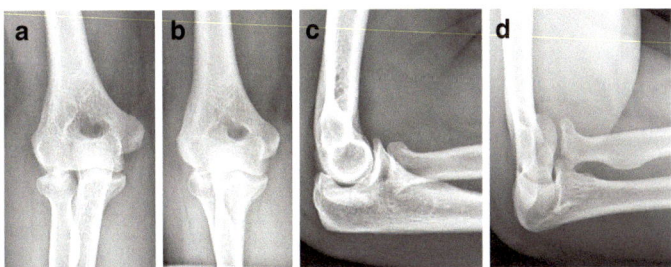

FIGURE 7.1 Pre-operative radiographs of a 44 year-old male patient with a comminuted displaced right radial head fracture with an associated mechanical block determined to be Grade III on intraoperative assessment. (**a**). AP view, (**b**). AP pronated view, (**c**). Lateral view, (**d**). Radial head view

Mason described the original classification system including type I, II, and III fractures of the radial head (Fig. 7.2) [6]. This was later modified by Johnston to include a fourth type, associated with elbow dislocation [7]. Broberg and Morrey modified the Mason classification to better guide treatment, and their system is most commonly used in the literature. Type I fractures have intra-articular displacement <2 mm. Type II fractures are displaced >2 mm or angulated and Type III fractures are comminuted and displaced fractures of the radial head [8].

While certain algorithms are largely accepted in the treatment of radial head fractures (Table 7.1), gold standards are not firmly established. Patients who present with minimally displaced fractures (<2 mm) and do not have a mechanical block to motion may be treated nonoperatively. Typical nonoperative protocols include a brief period of immobilization in a sling. After 1 week, active range of motion is begun with physical therapy. Immobilization should be discontinued by 4 weeks. If by 6 weeks patients exhibit loss of full extension, static progressive night splinting may be initiated.

Those fractures that are significantly displaced have a concomitant injury, or those with a mechanical block to motion should be considered for surgical fixation. Surgical treatment options include open reduction internal fixation (ORIF), radial head replacement, and less commonly fragment excision or radial head excision. In preparation for surgery

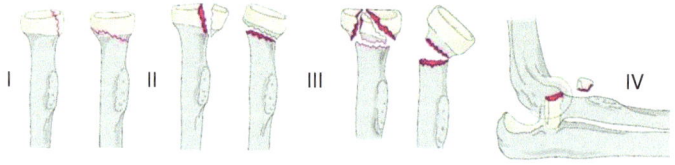

FIGURE 7.2 Mason classified radial head fractures as nondisplaced, displaced, and displaced and comminuted [6]. Johnston added a fourth type, which entails all radial head fractures in concomitance with an elbow dislocation. (From Eygendaal [18] with permission)

TABLE 7.1 Treatment algorithm of radial head fractures

Radial head fracture treatment algorithm		
Nondisplaced		Nonoperative
Displaced	No block to motion or associated injury	Nonoperative
	Small unrepairable fragments	Fragment excision
	Three or less repairable fragments	Open reduction internal fixation
	Large unrepairable fragments	Radial head arthroplasty
	Large unrepairable fragments with maintained stability in low demand patient	Radial head excision

the physician should be ready to perform ORIF or radial head replacement. Appropriate implants and hardware for both procedures should be present prior to the start of the case. It may be useful to utilize a headlamp during surgery to aid in visualization.

The patient is positioned supine with a bump under the ipsilateral scapula and a nonsterile arm tourniquet is placed. Prior to draping, fluoroscopic images should be obtained to confirm adequate visualization and appropriate patient positioning. At the time of surgery, intraoperative stress examinations should be performed to assess the competency of the medial and lateral ligament complexes with varus and valgus stress tests, respectively. Once prepped, draped, and a tourniquet inflated after exsanguination, an oblique lateral skin incision is made over the radial head and lateral epicondyle about 5–7 cm in length. Superficial dissection is carried through either the Kocher or Kaplan interval. The Kocher interval may be chosen if the LUCL is already known to be disrupted (Fig. 7.3); otherwise the Kaplan is more favorable

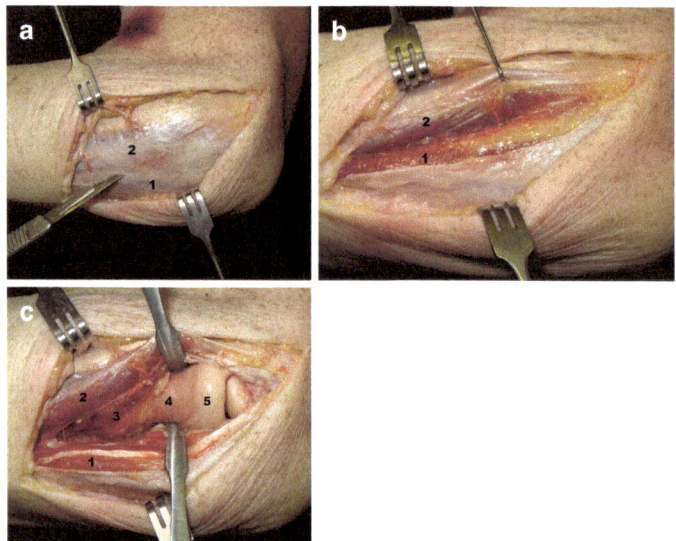

Figure 7.3 The Kocher approach. (**a**). Localize the "white line" and small perforator arteries to identify the interval between the anconeus and the extensor carpi ulnaris (ECU) muscle. It is easier to define this interval in the distal part of the approach. (**b**). Incision of the superficial aponeurosis and retraction of both muscles, anconeus and ECU muscles. (**c**). Open the capsule just anterior to the lateral ulnar collateral ligament. Exposition of the neck and the head of the radius. (1). Anconeus muscle, (2). ECU muscle, (3). Supinator muscle, (4). Neck of the radius, (5). Head of the radius. (From Barco et al. [19] with permission)

(Fig. 7.4). The downside to the Kaplan approach is the proximity of the posterior interosseous nerve (PIN) and the inability to extend the interval distally if needed. To protect the PIN, the forearm should be placed in pronation throughout dissection and exposure. A utilitarian posterior approach to the elbow can be used depending on the associated injuries involved. Tag sutures placed in the layered approach and in the proximal and distal stumps of the LCL can be useful for quick identification at the end of the case.

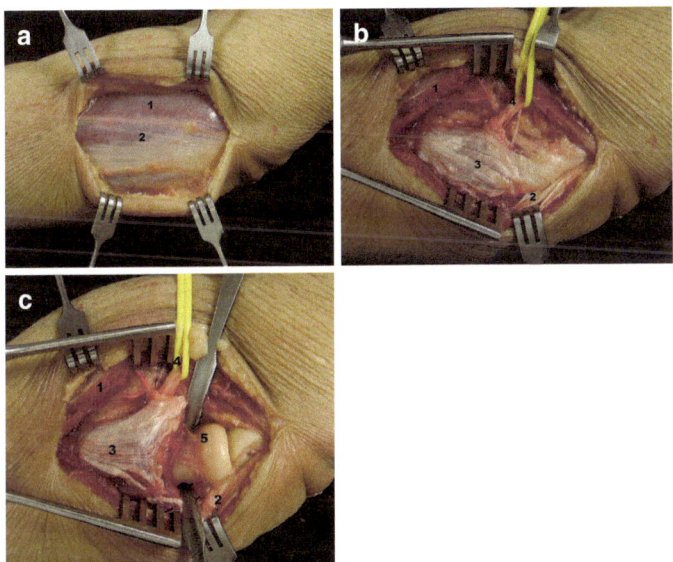

FIGURE 7.4 The Kaplan approach. (**a**). Superficial view of the proximal forearm. The incision is in line with the interval between the extensor carpi radialis brevis muscle and the extensor digitorum muscle. (**b**). It is necessary to elevate and retract this muscle in order to show the supinator muscle. Localize the key structure of the area, the radial nerve. With forearm pronation, the posterior interosseous nerve moves medially from the operative field. (**c**). Incise the annular ligament, the joint capsule, and the proximal origin of the supinator muscle to expose the capitellum and the radial head. (1). Extensor carpi radialis brevis muscle, (2). Extensor digitorum muscle, (3). Supinator muscle, (4). Radial nerve, posterior interosseous nerve, (5). Radial head. (From Barco et al. [19] with permission)

Once the radial head is identified it should be inspected for number of pieces, comminution, and their potential to accept fixation. Much of the radial head articulates with the proximal ulna but a "safe zone" for fixation occurs on the superolateral aspect. This non-articular segment has been noted to be a 110 degree arc centered on a point 10 degrees anterior to the midpoint of the lateral side of the radial head as judged in neutral rotation [9]. It can be identified intraoperatively based on its rounded appearance as opposed to the flat surface which articulates with the proximal ulna. Clinically this safe zone corresponds with the area between the radial styloid and Lister's tubercle. Open reduction and internal fixation (ORIF) should be attempted on displaced fractures that are repairable. Generally, two and three part fractures do well with ORIF [10, 11]. Conversely, it has been found that greater than three fragments have a higher failure rate with ORIF [12, 13]. Dissection should avoid extensive soft tissue stripping and all fragments should maintain their soft tissue attachments if possible. Dissection should be avoided posteriorly to protect the LUCL if the Kaplan interval is utilized. Provisional fixation can be achieved with K wires. Final fixation can be obtained with cannulated headless compression screws, bioabsorbable pins, or plates if necessary. When using screw fixation one should avoid perforation of the far cortex to prevent irritation of the proximal radioulnar joint (PRUJ) postoperatively. All screws should be countersunk. Hardware should be placed in the "safe zone" mentioned above. Plate fixation should be used only if other methods are unable to maintain fixation as it is more likely to damage the pericervical arterial blood supply [14]. Plate fixation may become symptomatic postoperatively and require removal once fracture union has been achieved.

In circumstances where the radial head cannot be repaired, there are more than three fragments, or a radial head resection is contraindicated, a radial head arthroplasty is indicated. The surgical approach is identical to what has been described for ORIF. When removing the radial head, it is ideal to keep fragments associated as much as possible. The neck cut should be made with an oscillating saw while protecting the surrounding soft tissue. Using Homan or baby Bennet retractors to expose the proximal radial diaphysis can be extremely beneficial for neck cut and component implantation. The removed radial head should be sized on the back table for diameter and thickness. The implant diameter should be sized to match the minor diameter of the native head. Regarding thickness, the proximal aspect of the implant should articulate with the PRUJ, which is anatomically 2 mm distal to the coronoid [15]. It is imperative to not simply fill the lateral joint space as the LCL is often torn causing more room than would normally be present. Implants that are too large can lead to pain and subsequent degeneration of articulating surfaces. After implantation, intraoperative inspection of elbow range of motion and the DRUJ, including fluoroscopic evaluation of ulnar variance, should be performed. The IOM can be assessed with longitudinal traction on the intact radial neck with attention placed to the ulnar variance under fluoroscopy.

At the completion of ORIF or arthroplasty the incision should be closed in layers. Capsular tissue, LCL, fascia and skin should all be closed individually. The integrity of the LUCL is imperative and if a humeral avulsion is present, repair should be performed to the isometric point of the humeral lateral epicondyle.

Certain fractures that are significantly displaced but not repairable may be indicated for fragment excision. It may be difficult to determine if a fragment is repairable preoperatively but advanced imaging with CT scans has helped with this significantly. Fragments that represent >25% of the articular surface are a contraindication to fragment excision [16]. Elbow arthroscopy may be especially useful for fragment excision as it can help to better visualize the joint and is associated with less soft tissue disruption compared to an open approach.

Even less commonly indicated is radial head resection. Certainly, some comminuted, nonrepairable fracture patterns may be indicated for resection. However, contraindications to this procedure are almost any concomitant injury, including MCL, LCL, IOM injuries, and elbow dislocations. In these instances, resection of the radial head can lead to significant instability and replacement may be a better option if fixation is not achievable. Resection may be performed for failed ORIF after recovery from the acute injury or patients with persistent pain from joint degeneration as delayed excision has been shown to be effective [17]. Radial head resection can be performed either open or arthroscopically. The annular ligament and LUCL should be maintained to prevent instability. The level of resection should go just distal to the radial notch. Regardless, radial head resection can place increased tension on the MCL and lead to posterolateral rotational instability. It is very rarely indicated in acute fractures.

Patients should be immobilized for 1–2 weeks postoperatively prior to beginning gentle range of motion. Restrictions in motion are dependent on associated injuries. Early motion is encouraged to avoid stiffness. Patients are allowed increased weight bearing at 6 weeks. Postoperative images should include AP and lateral radiographs (Fig. 7.5).

In summary, radial head fractures are common and choosing the correct treatment is critical to maximize outcomes. Several pearls to radial head fracture care can minimize the difficulty associated with surgical treatment (Table 7.2). The role of the radial head in elbow stability is central to this discussion. Associated injuries are common and should be accurately diagnosed and treated appropriately. Minimally displaced fractures without a mechanical block to motion can

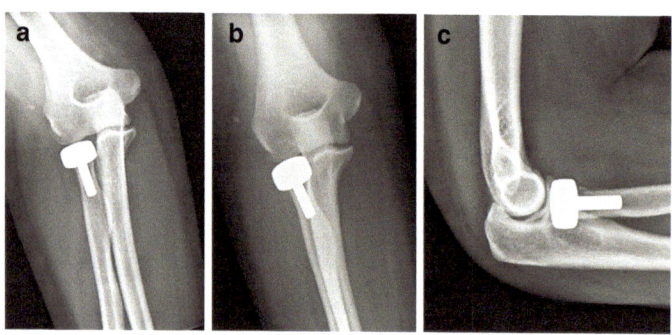

FIGURE 7.5 Postoperative radiographs of a 44 year-old male patient with a four-part Grade III radial head fracture with fragments determined to be unrepairable due to size and vascularity, treated with a right radial head arthroplasty. (**a**). AP view, (**b**). AP pronated view, (**c**). Lateral view. Preoperative images displayed in Fig. 7.1

TABLE 7.2 Authors' pearls

Authors' pearls
Perform a complete examination of the upper extremity with attention paid to neurovascular status, medial and lateral collateral ligaments, intraosseous membrane and DRUJ to evaluate for associated injuries
Utilize aspiration of hemarthrosis and injection of local anesthetic to assist in evaluation for mechanical block
Obtain appropriate imaging including radiographs and additional CT if necessary. Utilize two separate AP radiographs if warranted. Contralateral elbow images and DRUJ views can be useful for comparison
Individualize treatment based on patient, fracture, and injury characteristics including associated injuries
Be prepared by having hardware and implants available for both ORIF and arthroplasty
Utilize a headlamp to assist with visualization
Protect the PIN by maintaining forearm in pronated position throughout dissection and by performing subperiosteal dissection
Protect the LUCL throughout the procedure
Utilize tag stitches to assist in layered closure at the completion of the procedure
Utilize retractors to assist in exposure and to deliver the radial head and neck through the wound
Limit prominent hardware and attempt to keep hardware within the "safe zone"
Base the size of the radial head implant on the excised fracture fragments and PRUJ to limit the risk of overstuffing
Perform thorough intraoperative fluoroscopic examination of elbow and wrist, specifically DRUJ
Immobilize postoperatively for 1–2 weeks and then begin early range of motion, allowing increased weight bearing at 6 weeks

be treated with brief immobilization and early motion therapy. Open reduction internal fixation is ideal for non-comminuted displaced fractures with good success reported. Those fractures that are comminuted and displaced will likely benefit most from a radial head arthroplasty. Arthroplasty implants should always be available when treating radial head fractures as intraoperative findings may prevent successful repair. Radial head resection should be avoided in the acute setting secondary to the high incidence of associated injuries. Fragment excision may be ideal for isolated, displaced, small nonrepairable fragments. Radial head fracture care should be individualized based on the patient, fracture, and associated injuries to allow for the best outcomes.

References

1. Duckworth A, Clement N, Jenkins P, Aitken S, Court-Brown C. The epidemiology of radial head and neck fractures. J Hand Surg Am. 2012;37(1):112–9.
2. Kaas L, van Riet R, Vroemen J, Eygendaal D. The epidemiology of radial head fractures. J Shoulder Elbow Surg. 2010;19(4):520–3.
3. Halls A, Travill A. Transmission of pressures across the elbow joint. Anat Rec. 1964;150(3):243–7.
4. Greenspan A. Orthopedic imaging. 1st ed. Philadelphia: Wolters Kluwer/Lippincott, Williams & Wilkins; 2011.
5. Kaas L, van Riet R, Turkenburg J, Vroemen J, van Dijk C, Eygendaal D. Magnetic resonance imaging in radial head fractures: most associated injuries are not clinically relevant. J Shoulder Elbow Surg. 2011;20(8):1282–8.
6. Mason M. Some observations on fractures of the head of the radius with a review of one hundred cases. Br J Surg. 1954;42(172):123–32.
7. Johnston G. A follow-up of one hundred cases of fracture of the head of the radius with a review of the literature. Ulster Med J. 1962;31:51–6.
8. Broberg M, Morrey B. Results of treatment of fracture-dislocations of the elbow. Clin Orthop Relat Res. 1987;(216):109–19.

9. Smith G, Hotchkiss R. Radial head and neck fractures: anatomic guidelines for proper placement of internal fixation. J Shoulder Elbow Surg. 1996;5(2):113–7.

10. Lindenhovius A, Felsch Q, Ring D, Kloen P. The long-term outcome of open reduction and internal fixation of stable displaced isolated partial articular fractures of the radial head. J Trauma Inj Infect Crit Care. 2009;67(1):143–6.

11. Lindenhovius A, Felsch Q, Doornberg J, Ring D, Kloen P. Open reduction and internal fixation compared with excision for unstable displaced fractures of the radial head. J Hand Surg Am. 2007;32(5):630–6.

12. Ring D, Quintero J, Jupiter J. Open reduction and internal fixation of fractures of the radial head. J Bone Joint Surg. 2002;84A:1811–5.

13. Chen X, Wang S, Cao L, Yang G, Li M, Su J. Comparison between radial head replacement and open reduction and internal fixation in clinical treatment of unstable, multi-fragmented radial head fractures. Int Orthop. 2011;35(7):1071–6.

14. Koslowsky T, Schliwa S, Koebke J. Presentation of the microscopic vascular architecture of the radial head using a sequential plastination technique. Clin Anat. 2011;24(6):721–32.

15. Doornberg J, Linzel D, Zurakowski D, Ring D. Reference points for radial head prosthesis size. J Hand Surg Am. 2006;31(1):53–7.

16. Beingessner D, Dunning C, Gordon K, Johnson J, King G. The effect of radial head fracture size on elbow kinematics and stability. J Orthop Res. 2005;23(1):210–7.

17. Broberg M, Morrey B. Results of delayed excision of the radial head after fracture. J Bone Joint Surg Am. 1986;68(5):669–74.

18. Eygendaal D. Radial head fractures. In: Pederzini L, Eygendaal D, Denti M, editors. Elbow and sport. Berlin, Heidelberg: Springer; 2016.

19. Barco R, Ballesteros JR, Llusá M, Antuña S. Applied anatomy and surgical approaches to the elbow. In: Antuña S, Barco R, editors. Essentials in elbow surgery. London: Springer; 2014.

Chapter 8
Monteggia and Monteggia Variant Fractures

Michael Karl-Heinz Wich

Introduction

The classical Monteggia fracture dislocation was first described by Giovanni Battista Monteggia in 1814 as a proximal ulna fracture in combination with a dislocation of the radiocapitellar and the proximal radioulnar joint [1].

The term "Monteggia variant" refers to additional traumatic pathologies around the elbow (e.g., additional fractures of the radial head or dislocation of the humeroulnar joint). Dislocation of the proximal radioulnar joint (PRUJ) is a key characteristic which distinguishes this type of injury from other olecranon fractures [2]. Monteggia and Monteggia variants are rare injuries, representing about 2–5% of all proximal forearm fractures.

In 1967, Bado suggested a classification scheme respecting both the direction of radial head dislocation and the angulation of the ulnar fracture.

M. K.-H. Wich (✉)
Department of Trauma and Orthopedic Surgery,
Unfallkrankenhaus Berlin, Berlin, Germany

© Springer Nature Switzerland AG 2020   117
D. S. Horwitz et al. (eds.), *Tips and Tricks for Problem Fractures, Volume I*,
https://doi.org/10.1007/978-3-030-38274-2_8

Classification

Bado Type I lesions are highly prevalent in children and must be treated according to pediatric trauma principles (including closed reduction with casting, closed ECMES nailing, and open reduction with plating) [3, 4].

Bado Type I: Fractures with extension angulation within the proximal ulna fracture and anterior dislocation of the radial head (Fig. 8.1).

While only 15% of all Monteggia fracture dislocations are classified as Bado Type II, they dominate adult fractures (70–80%).

Bado Type II: Fractures with flexion angulation within the proximal ulna fracture and posterior dislocation of the radial head (Fig. 8.2).

Given the high prevalence of Bado Type II Monteggia lesions in adults, Jupiter suggested a sub-classification of the Bado scheme (type IIA to IID) for a stratified management (Fig. 8.3).

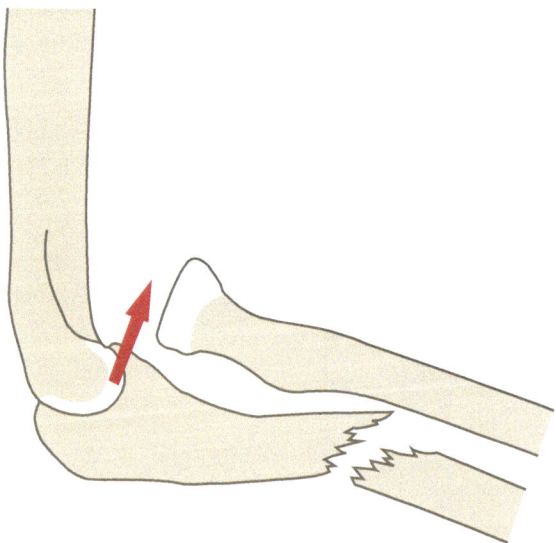

FIGURE 8.1 Monteggia fracture dislocation, Bado Type I

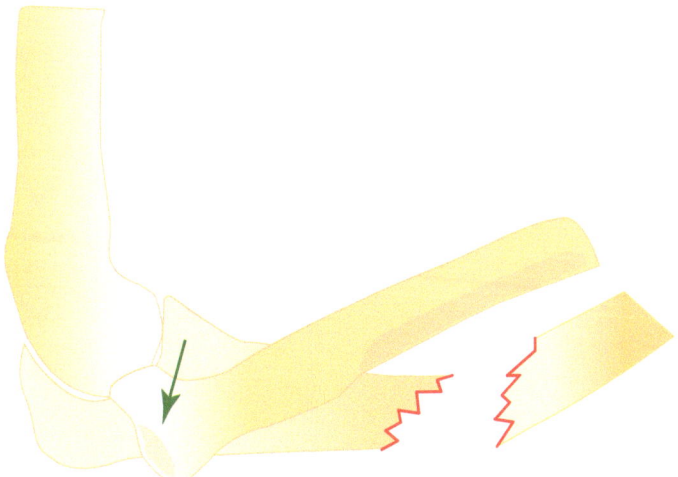

FIGURE 8.2 Monteggia fracture dislocation, Bado Type II

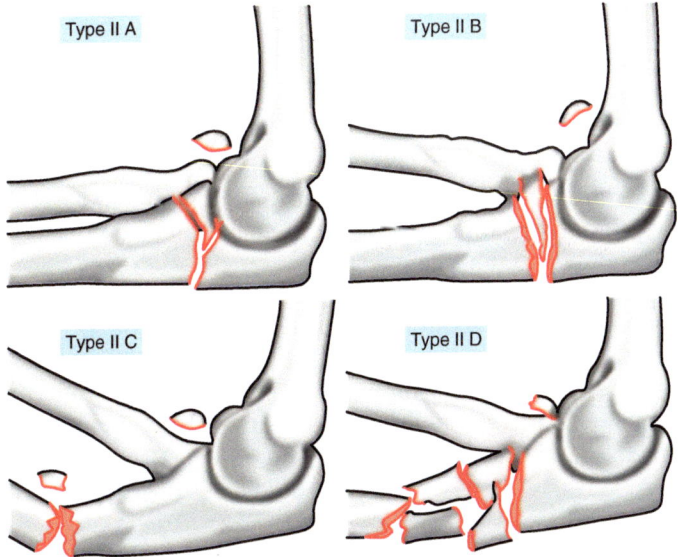

FIGURE 8.3 Monteggia fracture dislocation, Bado Type II, sub-classification by Jupiter, Type IIA, IIB, IIC and IID

FIGURE 8.4 Monteggia
fracture dislocation,
Bado Type III

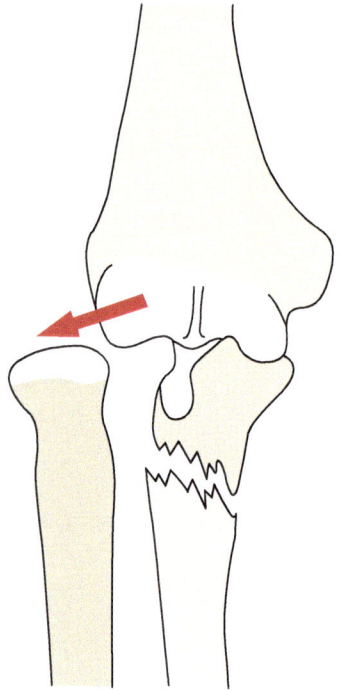

With three compromised joints and adjacent soft tissues,
Monteggia fracture dislocations demand meticulous reduction and fixation techniques.

Bado Type III: Fractures with valgus angulation within the
proximal ulna fracture and lateral dislocation of the radial
head (Fig. 8.4).

Bado Type IV: Fractures of the proximal ulna and radius
together with an anterior dislocation of the radial head
(Fig. 8.5).

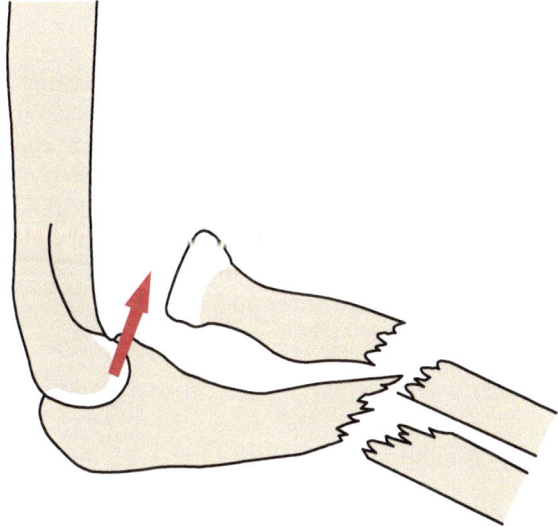

FIGURE 8.5 Monteggia fracture dislocation, Bado Type IV

Diagnosis

Postero-anterior and medial- lateral plain radiographs remain the standard of care for diagnosing and classifying fractures around the elbow. Although rare, radiographs must rule out an Essex-Lopresti lesion (i.e., a fracture of the radial head with concomitant dislocation of the distal radio-ulnar joint and disruption of the interosseous membrane). Thus, apart from the elbow joint, radiographs must also depict the forearm and the wrist. For a thorough evaluation of the fracture and dislocation (subluxation) pattern, precise projections are essential. In cases of suspected intra-articular fragments, radial head fractures, fracture reaching into the elbow joint (Jupiter Type IIA) or multiple fragments of the proximal ulna, computed tomography (CT) is warranted.

Preoperative Planning

Careful preoperative planning is the key to successful surgery. Understanding the fracture and recognizing associated injuries will allow the surgeon to appropriately plan the procedure and ensure that all necessary equipment and hardware is available.

Positioning of the patient and choosing the proper approach may determine the success or failure of surgery, and both must be determined based on the fracture pattern and bony and soft-tissue structures involved.

Patient Positioning

The setup for the surgical procedure is an important first important step because this will provide sufficient access to the proximal forearm and the elbow joint if chosen correctly (Figs. 8.6, 8.7, and 8.8).

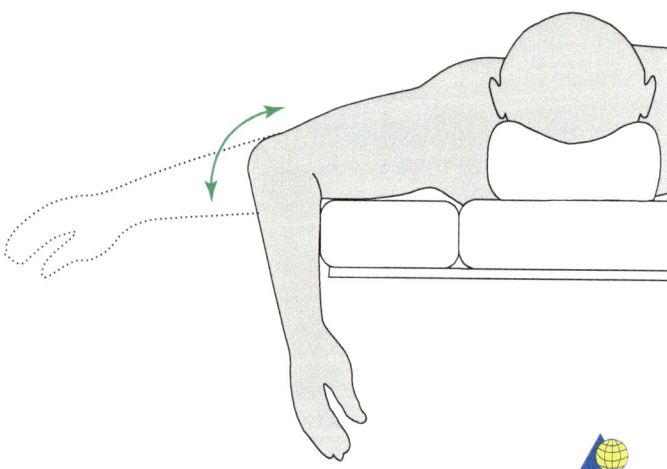

FIGURE 8.6 Patient positioning: prone position

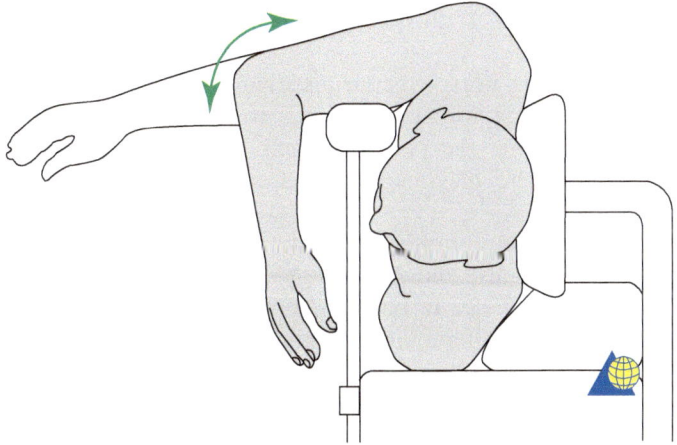

FIGURE 8.7 Patient positioning: lateral decubitus position

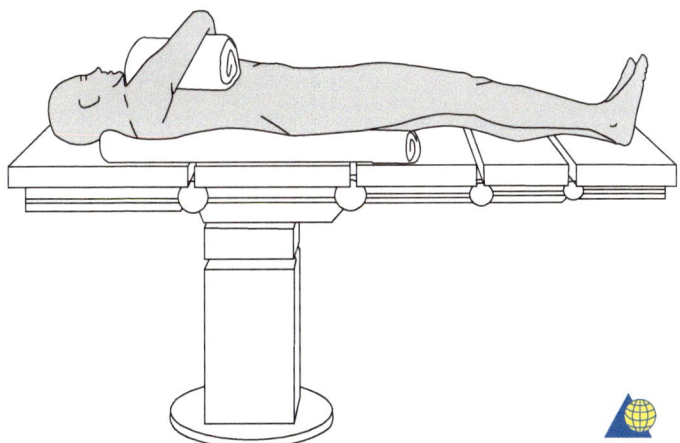

FIGURE 8.8 Patient positioning: supine position

Surgical Approach

The "working horse" for all proximal ulna, olecranon, and trans-olecranon forearm fractures is the posterior midline approach along the palpable ulnar bone ridge proximally leading to the olecranon and, if necessary, to the distal humerus [5].

This incision not only provides access to the ulna and the olecranon but also allows for reaching the radial head and the coronoid tubercle. It poses less risk to cutaneous nerve branches than other medial or lateral approaches.

A seperate incision and Kocher approach may be needed for reconstructing the radial head while lifting the lateral aspect of the full-thickness skin flap. A medial Hotchkiss approach may be required to reattach fragments of the coronoid (Fig. 8.9).

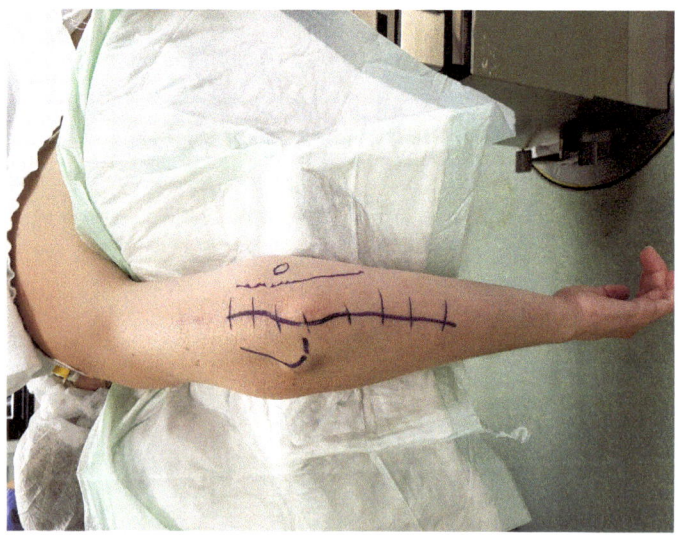

FIGURE 8.9 Prone position and posterior midline approach

Surgical Principles

Joint Reconstruction Without Remaining Steps and Gaps in the Articular Surface

If there is a concomitant radial head fracture in a Monteggia fracture dislocation when do you address the radial head, and how?

After exposing the proximal ulna fracture, the surgeon should try to access the radial head through the mobilized ulna fragments around the proximal radio-ulnar joint. Sometimes the access to the radial head is easy especially when there is comminution of the proximal ulna and the fragment that holds the crista supinatoris is mobile.

If this is not feasible, an additional Kocher approach (through the same extended skin incision) should be performed.

Small flake fractures that cannot be fixed should be removed from the joint at that time.

We recommend in Monteggia fracture dislocations not to resect the radial head without replacing it with a radial head prosthesis. The reason for this is that a resection adds a substantial amount of instability in an already unstable situation.

The younger the patient the more we try to preserve the radial head. In our hand even an "on table" reconstruction and plate fixation is a good technique. In some patients this radial head will only function as a spacer due to partial necrosis or non-union. Still, later on, after the fracture of the ulna has uneventfuly healed, a resection or a replacement of the radial head can be done with much better outcome.

Force distribution between the medial and the lateral part of the elbow is different. Sixty percent of all forces that are transferred via the elbow joint are located at the radiocapitellar joint and, therefore, show the importance of the radial part of the joint for stability and force transmission (Fig. 8.10).

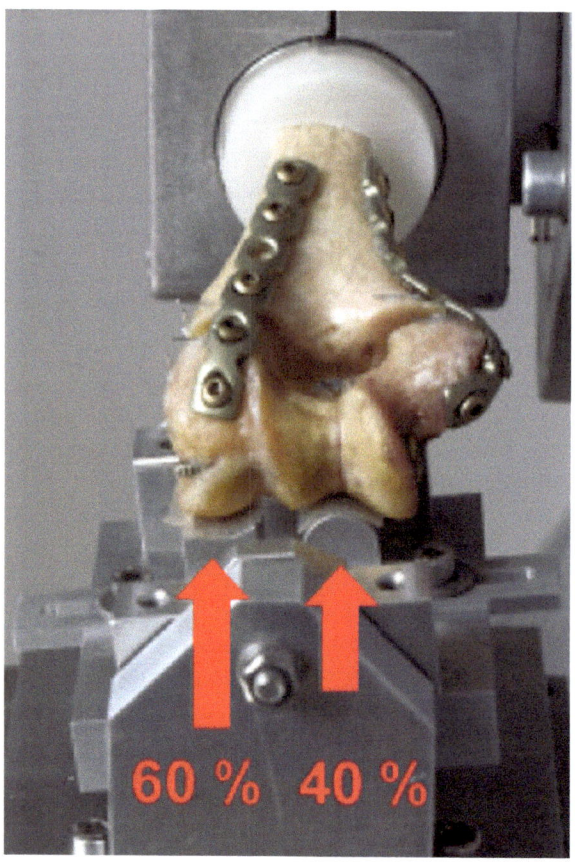

FIGURE 8.10 Typical force distribution between radial and ulnar columns of the distal humerus

Restoration of the Anatomical Axis of the Proximal Ulna and the Radius

This is a very important but difficult step of the procedure. In situations where the fracture of the proximal ulna is comminuted the first obstacle can be determining the correct length of the ulna to be restored.

The intact or reconstructed radial head gives the surgeon the best indication of the overall length of the forearm.

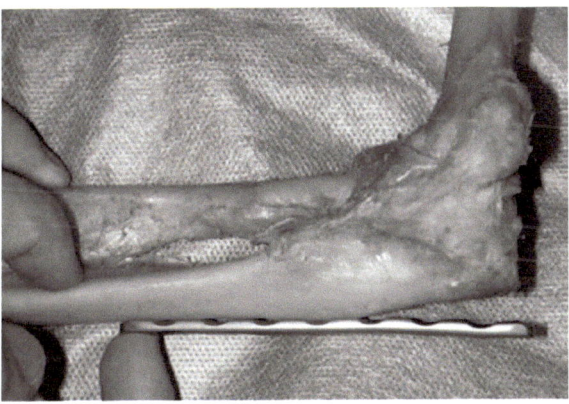

Visualization of the anterior deviation of the proximal ulna in comparison to a straight plate

Although we still use many straight plates to fix the proximal ulna, the ulna is not a straight bone (Fig. 8.11).

In the medial-lateral view of the proximal ulna, there is an individual but substantial anterior deviation which cannot be respected if using a straight plate. The ulnar plate has to be bent in order to maintain a centered alignment between radial head and capitellum (Figs. 8.12a and 8.14a).

In this patient the anterior deviation has been increased substantially through the fracture displacement, and this is obviously due to the fact that the axis of the radial shaft is no longer directed at the center of the capitellum and instead aims too distally (Fig. 8.12a).

Intraoperative c-arm pictures show the decrease in anterior angulation and the realignment of the radial shaft axis aiming again at the center of the capitellum after the surgical procedure (Fig. 8.12b).

The long intramedullary homerun screw adds stability to the construct.

The anterior deviation (bending) of the proximal ulna differs from 1° to 14° with a mean angle of 4,5° [6] (Fig. 8.13).

Posterior view of a left elbow joint. The white line displays the varus angulation of the proximal third of the ulna.

The varus angulation of the proximal third ulna is on average 17.5° (11–23°). A straight plate it is very difficult to bend

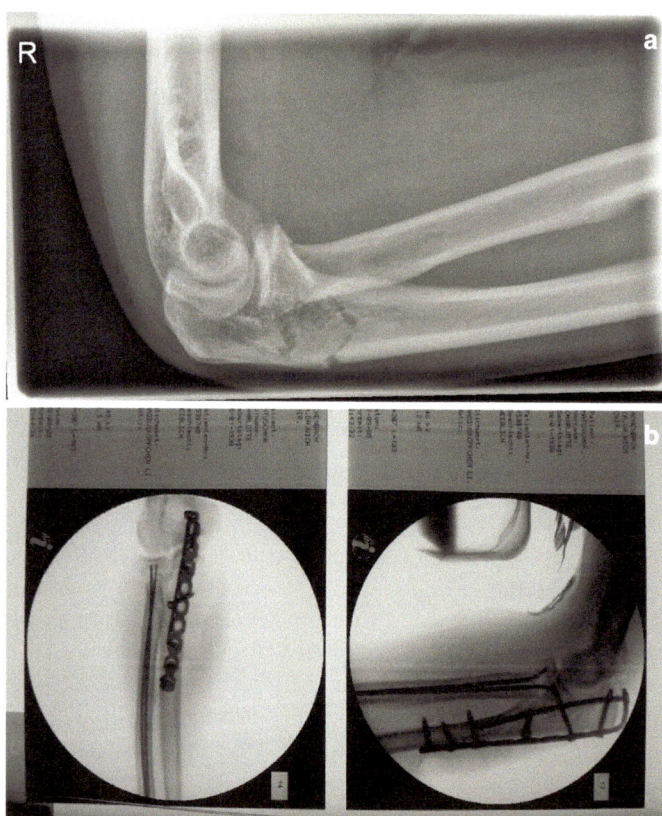

FIGURE 8.12 (**a**) Increased anterior deviation through fracture displacement. (**b**): Same patient as in (**a**), intraop c-arm x-rays with restoration of the anterior deviation of the proximal ulna and realignment of the radial shaft axis and the center of the humeral capitellum

to match the normal varus angulation, and although modern anatomically contoured implants match the varus they still must be individualized to the specific anatomy of each patient.

In situations where larger fragments can be reduced to their anatomic position, restoration of the axis and the spe-

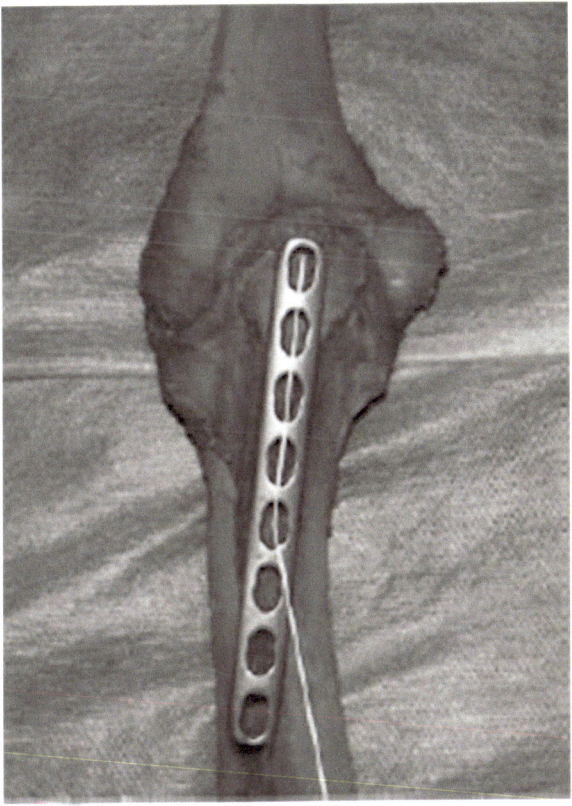

FIGURE 8.13 Varus angulation of the proximal ulna (white line) in comparison to a straight plate

cific angles of the ulna will not be a problem. In situations where the surgeon is confronted with a multifragment and comminuted fracture, standardized x-rays from the contralateral forearm can be helpful.

A reduction technique which can be helpful in these cases is to use a 2,5 mm K-wire or an ECMES-nail introduced through the olecranon beneath the subchondral bone of the joint line, bridging the fracture site and anchoring in the intact ulna shaft.

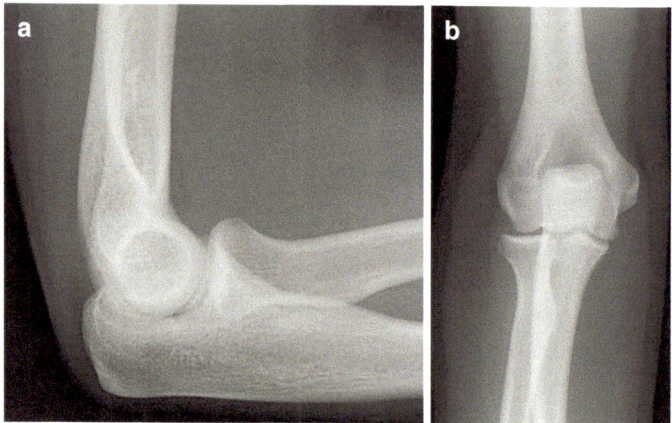

FIGURE 8.14 (**a**): Axis of the proximal radius meets the center of the humeral capitellum in medial-lateral x-ray plane. (**b**): Axis of the proximal radius meets the center of the humeral capitellum in anterior-posterior x-ray plane

With the bendable K-wire, anterior deviation and ulnar angulation can easily be corrected while the main fragments are preliminarily fixed to each other.

Before osteosynthesis is considered finished, the surgeon has to make sure that

- In both standard planes in the c-arm view the proximal radial shaft axis aims at the center of the capitellum (Fig. 8.14a, b), and a free range of motion has been established for extension and flexion in the elbow joint as well as pronation and supination of the forearm
- In the ap view the joint line of the humero-ulnar joint looks congruent and parallel (Fig. 8.14b)
- In the lateral view the trochlea humeri sits in the center of the semilunar notch of the ulnar and the joint space is over the whole circumference even and parallel
- No screw is crossing any of the joints and no screw blocks the free movement between ulna and radius during pronation and supination
- Free range of motion during extension/flexion and pronation and supination is achieved

Stability of the Osteosynthesis

Modern 3.5 and 4.0 plates with preshaped anatomical designs provide enough stability for the proximal ulna and the huge lever arm forces that will be produced through early functional treatment.

The length of the plate is still a critical factor, and we recommend the use of plates that proximally extend around the olecranon to allow a so-called home run screw to bridge the fracture site and add intramedullary stability to the plate. Distal to the ulna fracture the plate should be long enough to take at least four screws. (Figs. 8.15, 8.16, and 8.17)

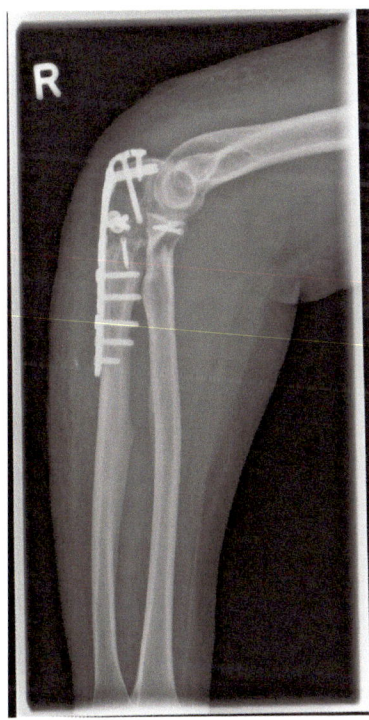

FIGURE 8.15
Biomechanically insufficient construct. The home run screw ends in the fracture zone; this led to a nonunion

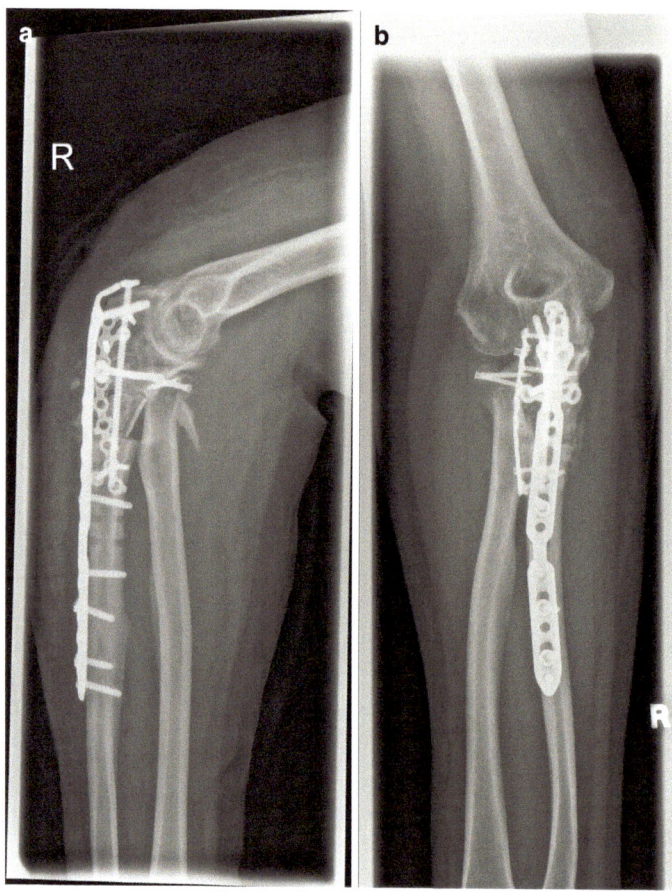

FIGURE 8.16 (**a**, **b**): Same patient as in Fig. 8.15 after nonunion and revision of the osteosynthesis with autologous bone (iliac crest)

The ulna fracture has healed after resection of the nonunion and interposition of a tricortical bone graft from the iliac crest an additional lateral 2.5 mm plate and a homerun screw crossing the former nonunion site were added to the construct.

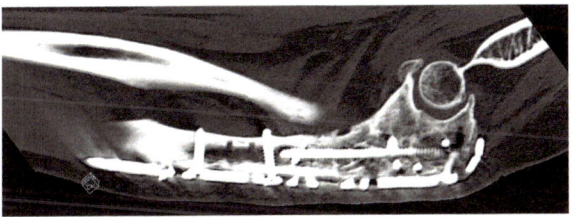

FIGURE 8.17 Same patient as in Figs. 8.15 and 8.16a, b. CT scan displaying full bony consolidation of former nonunion region

In cases where there is an extended area of a fracture comminution in the proximal ulna you can expect relevant torsion forces especially when the patient performs pronation and supination. In these circumstances we recommend the use of an additional smaller 2.5 or 2.7 mm plate at a 90° angle to the first plate (positioned medial or lateral to the posterior ridge).

Stability of the ulnar osteosynthesis is paramount in preventing the development of a nonunion and allowing early movement in order to obtain a good functional outcome.

Stability of the Joint

After reconstructing the articular surfaces of the radial head, the ulnar, and the radioulnar joint, and after accomplishing a stable osteosynthesis of the proximal ulna it is mandatory to check for axial alingement and joint stability.

At the end of the operation the surgeon should examine the elbow joint under fluoroscopy in extension, with varus and valgus stress to make sure that no excessive joint gaping will appear, indicating a major instability.

In full extension the joint should be stable with no signs of a subluxation (incongruency of the joint lines).

The surgeon should also perform the lateral pivot shift test when passively supinating the forearm under valgus stress; if the radial head dislocates out of the radiocapitellar joint this should be addressed by repairing the lateral ulnar collateral ligament (LUCL).

In severely unstable elbow joints an external hinged fixator helps to maintain the joint congruency and stills allows for postop movement of the joint.

Rehabilitation

The patient's arm is placed into a splint with the elbow in 90 degrees of flexion and the forearm in neutral position for 24–48 hours. Early active range of motion can start when the wound is stable.

A resting splint in the position of maximal stability may be beneficial between exercises. For patients requiring a lateral ligament repair, a protocol involving active flexion and extension in pronation should be instituted. The patient may supinate with the arm flexed to 90 degrees or beyond. Varus stress should be avoided at all times.

References

1. Andjelković S, et al. Giovanni Battista Monteggia (1762–1815). Srp Arh Celok Lek. 2015;143(1–2):105–7.
2. Rehim SA, Maynard MA, Sebastin SJ, Chung KC. Monteggia fracture-dislocations: a historical review. J Hand Surg Am. 2014;39(7):1384–94.
3. Bae DS. Successful strategies for managing Monteggia injuries. J Pediatr Orthop. 2016;36 Suppl 1:S67–70.
4. Slongo T, Fernandez FF. Incorrectly healed Monteggia lesion in childhood and adolescence. Unfallchirurg. 2011;114(4):311–22.
5. Dowdy PA, Bain GI, King GJ, Patterson SD. The midline posterior elbow incision. An anatomical appraisal. J Bone Joint Surg Br. 1995;77:696–9.
6. Grechenig W, Clement H, Pichler W, Tesch NP, Windisch G. The influence of lateral and anterior angulation of the proximal ulna on the treatment of a Monteggia fracture: an anatomical cadaver study. J Bone Joint Surg Br. 2007;89:836–8.

Chapter 9
Fractures of the Distal Radius

Daniela Sanchez, Daniel S. Horwitz, and Hemil Maniar

Case Presentation

A 56-year-old, right-hand-dominant woman sustained a fall from standing height and landed on her outstretched right hand. She arrived at the emergency room complaining of immediate pain, swelling, and deformity of the wrist. On exam she was found to have edema and severe pain with attempted range of motion. She had no distal neurovascular deficit. Wrist x-rays were taken (Fig. 9.1) and revealed a comminuted and impacted distal radius fracture with intra-articular extension and a displaced fracture of the ulnar styloid.

D. Sanchez · H. Maniar (✉)
Musculoskeletal Institute, Geisinger Health System,
Danville, PA, USA
e-mail: hmaniar@geisinger.edu

D. S. Horwitz
Department of Orthopaedic Surgery, Geisinger Health System,
Geisinger Musculoskeletal Institute, Danville, PA, USA

© Springer Nature Switzerland AG 2020   135
D. S. Horwitz et al. (eds.), *Tips and Tricks for Problem Fractures, Volume I*,
https://doi.org/10.1007/978-3-030-38274-2_9

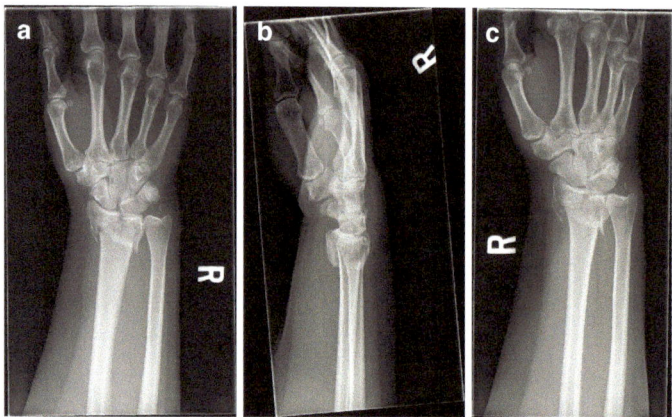

FIGURE 9.1 (**a–c**): Anteroposterior (AP), lateral, and oblique views of the right wrist – Injury films

In the emergency department, under a hematoma block, the patient underwent closed reduction and the extremity was splinted in a sugar tong splint. This is our routine practice, although there is now evidence to support splinting without a reduction without any increased adverse outcomes if decision to pursue surgery has already been made [1].

For definitive treatment, in addition to the fracture pattern and the assessment of the post-reduction fracture stability, patient specific factors such as their age, baseline functional activity, and treatment goals should be considered. In young patients, the functional outcomes correlate with the quality of fracture reduction and therefore surgical treatment may be preferred. Associated fractures of the ipsilateral limb or fractures of distant sites also need to be considered for decision making.

On the other hand, non-operative treatment has proven to be successful for older patients who do not have a high functional demand. The current literature does not support the theory that operative management can provide better clinical outcomes for elderly patients with distal radius fractures. Operative management can offer better radiographic outcomes and grip strength than nonsurgical treatment; however, the risk of complications requiring surgical treatment is greater. Thus, indications for operative fixation should be considered carefully in the treatment of the elderly [2].

In general, operative fixation of distal radius fracture is recommended in fracture patterns that are inherently unstable with subluxation or dislocation of the radiocarpal joint, open fractures, palmer metaphyseal comminution, significant radial shortening more than 3 mm, residual dorsal tilt of more than 10 degrees, significant dorsal comminution, and high-energy injuries which are inherently more unstable in a cast. Also, surgical treatment is recommended in patients with acute carpal tunnel syndrome.

The patient in the case presented above is otherwise healthy, works at a daycare managing more than 10 kids, is right hand dominant, and has a high functional demand. Based on patient characteristics and fracture pattern a decision was made to offer her surgical treatment. A volar locked plate construct was chosen to be the most appropriate for this fracture pattern.

Other techniques for operative fixation include dorsal plate fixation, k-wiring, external fixation, bridge plating, and fragment-specific fixation which are less commonly used and are beyond the scope of this chapter.

Preoperative Planning

When planning the surgical procedure, the main fracture fragments-radial styloid, dorso-ulnar, and palmar-ulnar fragments, should be identified. In cases with intra-articular extension, especially if there is comminution, a CT (computed tomography) scan can help to better understand the fracture pattern and aid in choosing the most appropriate surgical approach and fixation construct. A CT scan can also be beneficial for evaluating dorsal comminution, identifying the number of fragments, and assessing the integrity of the intermediate column and the sigmoid notch.

In this case a CT scan was performed (Fig. 9.2). The coronal cuts (Fig. 9.2a) show metaphyseal comminution and two main fracture fragments corresponding to the radial styloid and an ulnar corner. The sagittal cuts (Fig. 9.2b) show the degree of dorsal comminution. An axial CT cut (Fig. 9.2c) shows radial styloid, dorsal-ulnar, and volar-ulnar fragments.

The goals of surgical treatment are to reconstruct the biomechanics of the radial, intermediate and ulnar columns, achieve articular congruity, and allow the patient a prompt

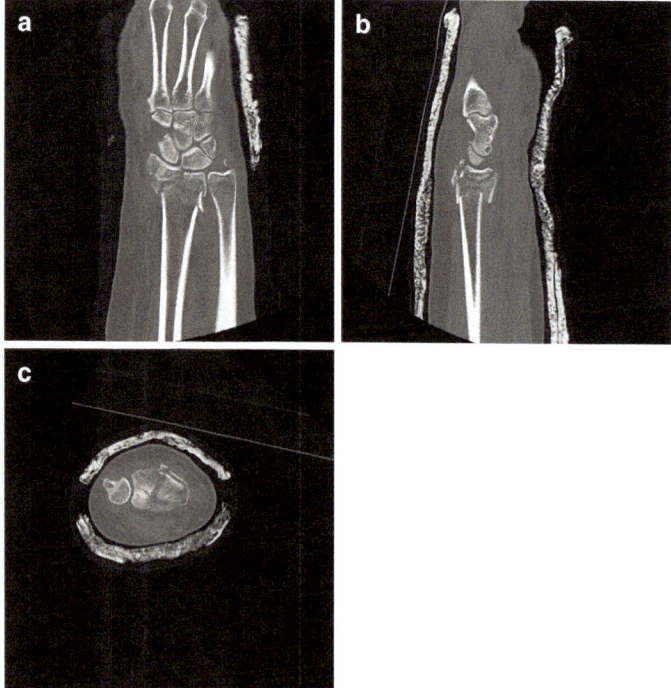

FIGURE 9.2 (**a–c**): Coronal, sagittal, and axial CT cuts

return to baseline function. Radial length, volar tilt, and ulnar variance should be restored as failing to do so could lead to poor functional outcomes.

Operative Treatment

The patient is positioned supine on a standard operating table. A hand table is utilized for the case. A non-sterile tourniquet is placed to the proximal arm and is prepped out of the surgical field. Tourniquet is inflated prior to incision.

A sound surgical technique is necessary to avoid complications. Loupe magnification is an option. A standard volar Henry's approach is chosen. Incision is fashioned from the distal wrist crease proximally along the tendon of flexor carpi radialis (FCR). The length of the incision varies according to the fracture pattern. The fascia over the FCR tendon is incised and the tendon is now retracted ulnarly to protect the median nerve. Care is taken to identify and protect the palmer cutaneous branch of median nerve and the radial artery during deep dissection. The deep forearm fascia is incised underneath the FCR sheath to gain access to deep forearm flexors which are also retracted ulnarly. The pronator quadratus is now identified and released distally and radially to expose the fracture site. For more complex fractures, a release of the distal insertion of the brachioradialis is recommended to neutralize the deforming forces on the radial styloid.

The main fracture fragments are identified and reduced under direct vision. A bone holding clamp is used to correct the rotation of proximal fragment and to apply counter traction for reduction. Elevation of the ulnar corner fragment is performed by using a Freer elevator. Manipulation of the distal fragment is generally achieved by direct traction and ulnar deviation of the thumb. A dental pick or an intrafocal freer elevator can correct dorsal angulation of the distal fragment (Fig. 9.3a, b). A K-wire through the styloid and a horizontal subchondral K-wire can be used to maintain reduction

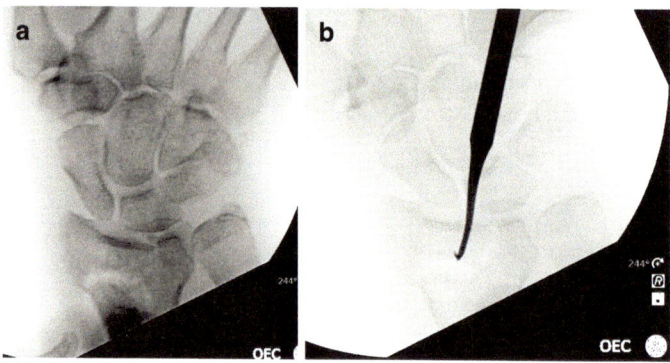

FIGURE 9.3 (**a**, **b**): Demonstrating use of a dental pick to fine tune articular reduction

before plate placement (Fig. 9.4). Very rarely, an external fixator with a distractor may be required. Adequacy of fracture reduction is assessed using AP (antero-posterior), lateral, lateral tilt, and oblique views.

A volar variable angle locking plate is positioned over the distal radius with care taken to place the plate proximal to the watershed line, which is the bony transverse ridge found along the volar distal edge of the radius that marks the distal extent of the concave-shaped pronator fossa. Position is checked under fluoroscopy. Multiple K-wires are used through holes in the plate to hold the plate to the bone. We place the K-wires in such a way that these serve as a guide for angulation of distal articular block locking screws (Fig. 9.5). The first screw is then placed in the oblong hole proximally; once the final position is confirmed, the plate is finally fixed with a combination of locking screws distally and locking/non-locking screws proximally.

Occasionally, the plate is used to correct residual volar tilt; in this case the plate is kept off the bone proximally and fixed distally. The volar tilt is restored once the proximal portion of the plate is reduced to the bone (Fig. 9.6). We usually insert the radial styloid screw in the end under fluo-

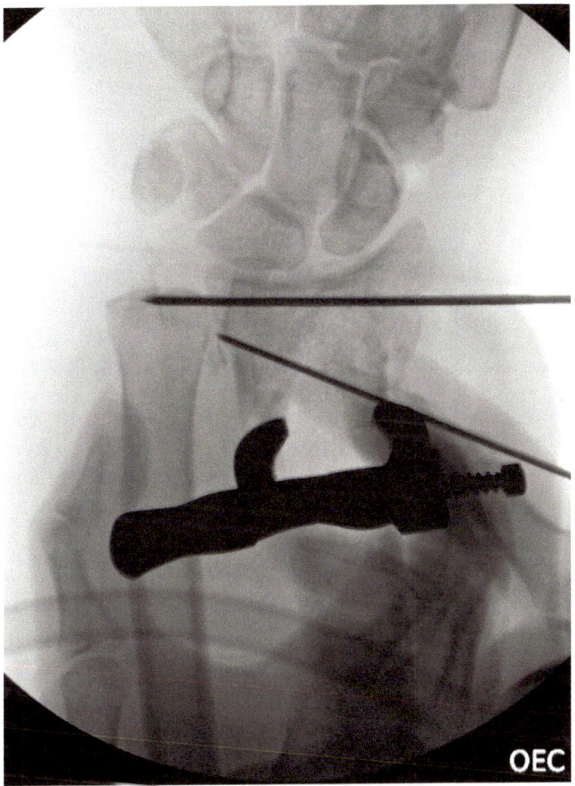

FIGURE 9.4 Subchondral K-wire used to hold the reduced ulnar corner articular piece

roscopy. Before insertion of this screw a true lateral of the joint is obtained to check for reduction as the radial styloid screw can block visualization. Distal screws are generally kept shorter (75%) to prevent tendon irritation [3]. Final images are taken including AP, lateral, oblique, and dorsal tangential views to check for final position of implants and adequacy of reduction (Fig. 9.7).

The tourniquet is deflated, and adequate hemostasis is ensured. After confirming good distal perfusion, the wound is

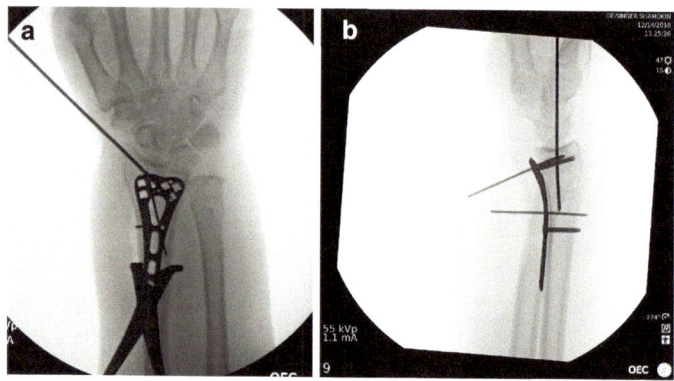

FIGURE 9.5 (**a, b**): Provisional plate placement with K-wires. Note the trajectory of the distal K-wire in lateral view. The distal articular screws are placed taking this wire into account to keep them extra-articular

irrigated. The pronator quadratus muscle is placed back to cover the plate, and the surgical wound is closed in a layered fashion.

Postoperative Protocol

Postoperatively, patients are splinted in a short arm volar plaster slab. Metacarpophalangeal joints are kept free. Patients are encouraged to mobilize their digits to decrease edema and are asked to start incorporating the extremity in activities to daily living while maintaining non-weight bearing precautions.

At the first follow up in 2 weeks, sutures are removed, and further immobilization is decided based on bone quality and fracture pattern. In keeping with recent literature, no x-rays are done at the first postoperative visit [4]. X-rays are taken at the 6-week follow-up visit at which time patients are mobilized with hand therapy. Final follow-up is at 3 months. Further follow-up is dependent on degree of recovery at final follow-up.

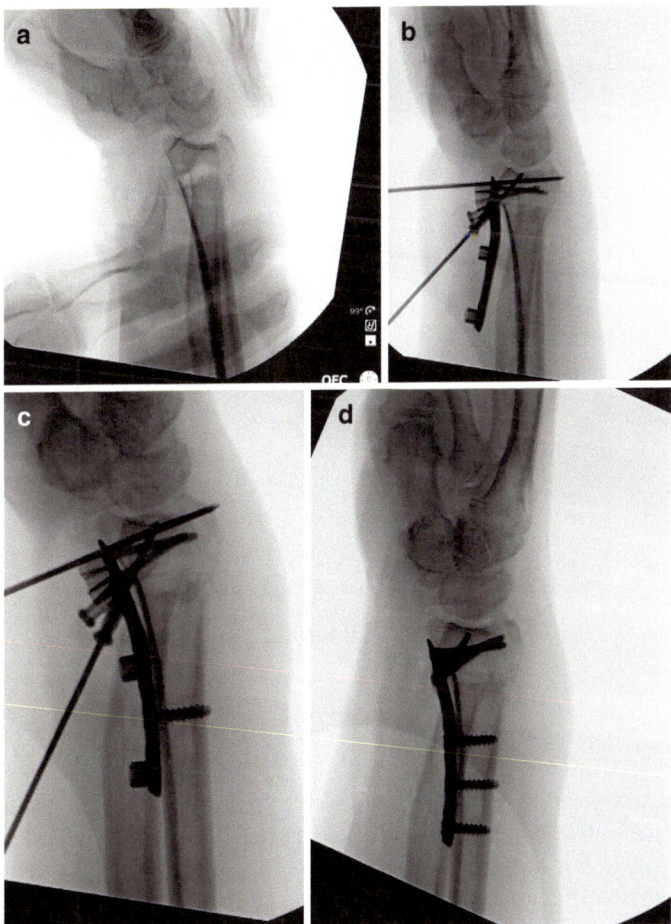

FIGURE 9.6 (**a**) Initial reduction, articular surface in neutral. (**b**) Distal part of the plate is fixed to the bone and proximal plate is off bone. (**c**) Proximal plate reduced to bone with cortical screw; note the return of volar tilt. (**d**) final construct in lateral plane

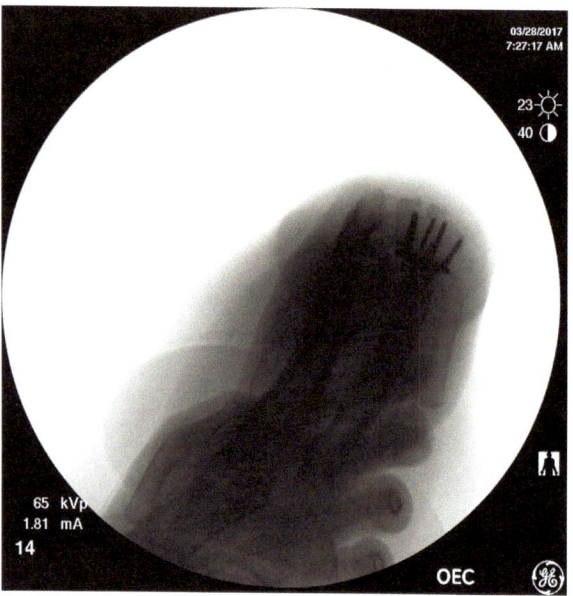

FIGURE 9.7 Tangential view showing distal articular screw lengths

Complications

Complications following operative treatment of distal radius are well known. These include but are not limited to infection, loss of fixation, nerve injury, complex regional pain syndrome, wrist stiffness, loss of grip strength, and arthritis. Volar locked plating, which has become the most popular choice of fixation in recent times, has been shown to be associated with 21 percent risk of need for secondary operations due to a complication [5, 6]. These typically include flexor tendon ruptures from a plate that is positioned too distally or extensor tendon ruptures from a dorsally penetrated screw tip.

References

1. Teunis T, Mulder F, Nota SP, Milne LW, Dyer GS, Ring D. No difference in adverse events between surgically treated reduced and unreduced distal radius fractures. J Orthop Trauma. 2015;29(11):521–5.
2. Chen Y, Chen X, Li Z, Yan H, Zhou F, Gao W. Safety and efficacy of operative versus nonsurgical management of distal radius fractures in elderly patients: a systematic review and meta-analysis. J Hand Surg Am. 2016;41(3):404–13.
3. Baumbach SF, Synek A, Traxler H, Mutschler W, Pahr D, Chevalier Y. The influence of distal screw length on the primary stability of volarplateosteosynthesis--a biomechanical study. J Orthop Surg Res. 2015;10:139.
4. Stone JD, Vaccaro LM, Brabender RC, Hess AV. Utility and cost analysis of radiographs taken 2 weeks following plate fixation of distal radius fractures. J Hand Surg Am. 2015;40(6):1106–9.
5. Williksen JH, Husby T, Hellund JC, Kvernmo HD, Rosales C, Frihagen F. External fixation and adjuvant pins versus volar locking plate fixation in unstable distal radius fractures: a randomized, controlled study with a 5-year follow-up. J Hand Surg Am. 2015;40(7):1333–40.
6. Lee DS, Weikert DR. Complications of distal radius fixation. Orthop Clin North Am. 2016;47(2):415–24.

Chapter 10
Scaphoid Fractures

Steven H. Goldberg

Illustrative Cases

Case 1: A 17-year-old female high school tennis player fell backwards and had acute right wrist pain. Initial radiographs were interpreted as normal (Fig. 10.1). She taped the wrist, wore a splint part-time, and finished her season. She presented 3.5 months postinjury with persistent 4/10 pain, a 7 degree loss of flexion, a 23 degree loss of extension, and a 12 pound decrease in grip strength compared to her other side.

Case 2: A 20-year-old female hairstylist was involved in an altercation and developed acute hand pain and suffered an acute small metacarpal neck fracture (Fig. 10.2). She noted wrist pain for 8 months duration secondary to a prior altercation in which radiographs were obtained and interpreted as normal. On exam she has snuffbox tenderness, small metacarpal tenderness, full finger motion, and wrist motion of 70 degrees in flexion and 50 degrees in extension.

S. H. Goldberg (✉)
Department of Orthopaedic Surgery, Geisinger Health System, Danville, PA, USA
e-mail: Steven.Goldberg@Bellin.org

© Springer Nature Switzerland AG 2020
D. S. Horwitz et al. (eds.), *Tips and Tricks for Problem Fractures, Volume I*,
https://doi.org/10.1007/978-3-030-38274-2_10

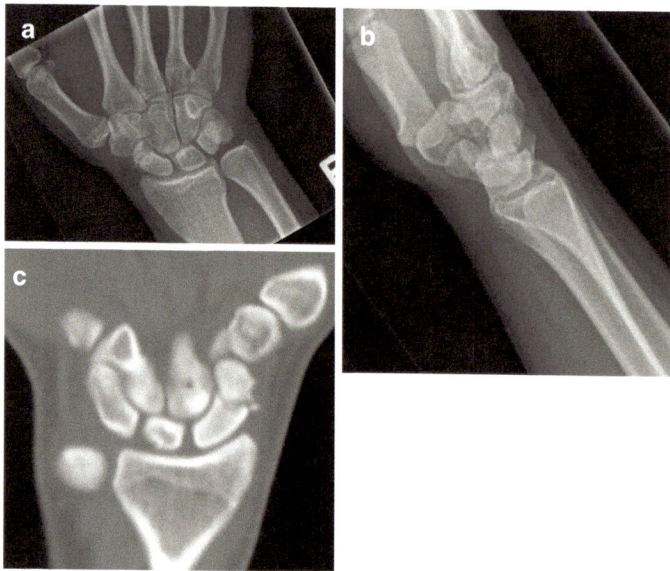

FIGURE 10.1 (a). PA radiograph 3.5 months post fall showing distal pole nonunion with some comminution. Note absence of radioscaphoid arthritis. (b). Lateral radiograph showing mild DISI deformity. (c). Coronal CT showing distal third fracture. (d). Sagittal CT showing fracture alignment. (e). Sagittal CT showing DISI deformity more clearly than lateral radiograph. (f). Intraoperative lateral fluoroscopy showing radiolunate joint pin with correction of DISI to neutral radio-lunate-capitate relationship. (g). PA fluoroscopy showing distal ulnar larger wire used as a distal pole joystick to manipulate the distal pole after radiolunate fixation. Central guide wire and anti-rotation wires also seen. (h). PA radiograph 10 weeks postop showing retrograde headless compression screw with healed fracture. Note increased density in radial styloid from bone graft substitute placement. (i). Lateral radiograph 10 weeks postop showing maintenance of neutral radio-lunate-capitate relationships. (j). Wrist flexion at 8 months. (k). Wrist extension at 8 months

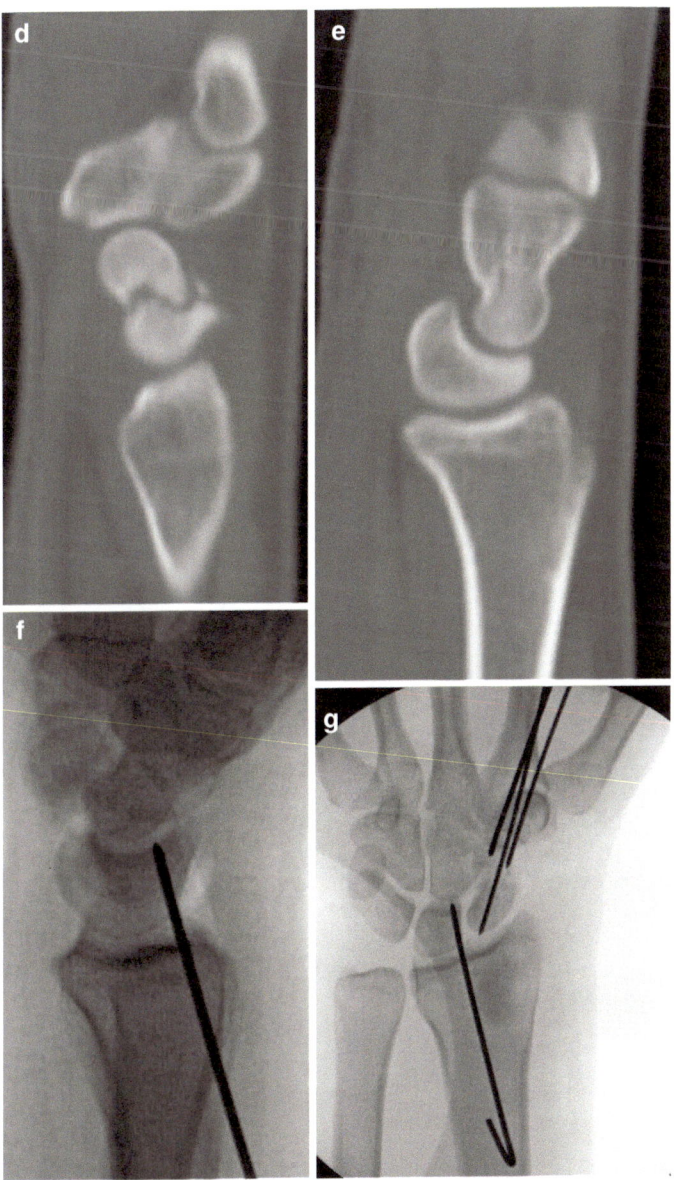

FIGURE 10.1 (continued)

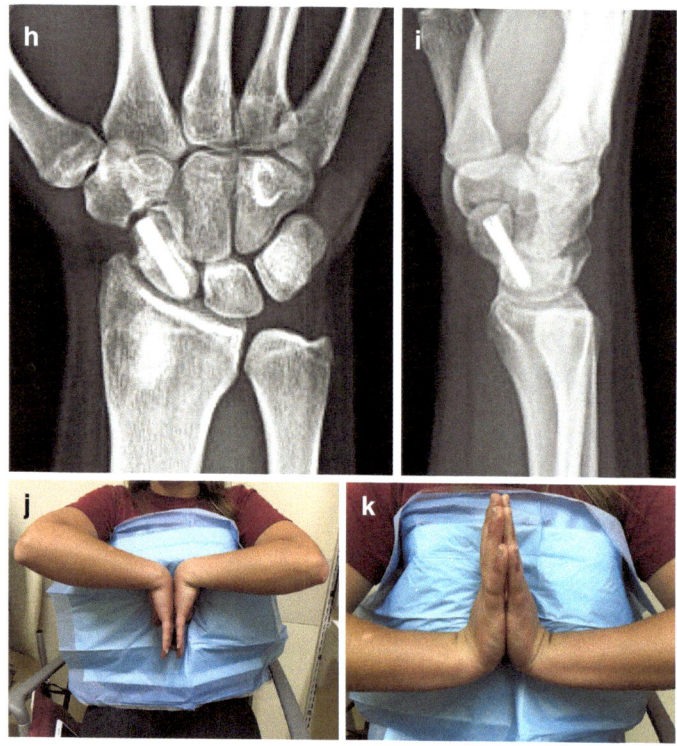

Figure 10.1 (continued)

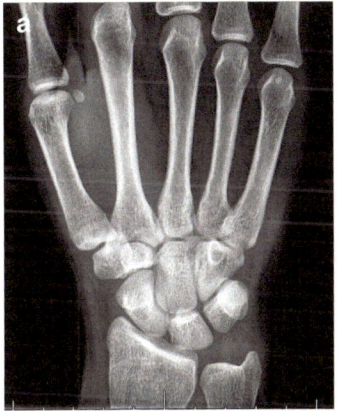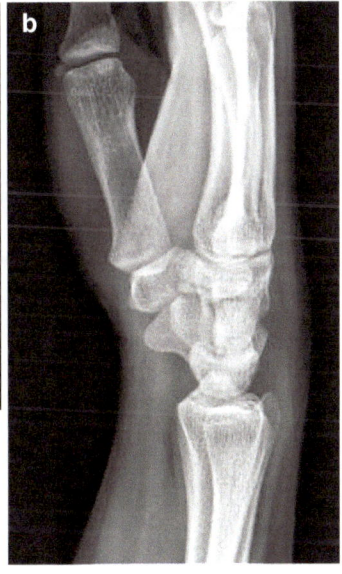

FIGURE 10.2 (**a**). PA initial view without clear fracture seen. (**b**). Lateral initial radiograph with no fracture seen and normal radio-lunate-capitate alignment. (**c**). Oblique initial radiograph showing a possible fracture line that was not initially appreciated by radiologist or emergency room provider. (**d**). Patient presents 8 months later with acute hand pain after punching a wall. A small metacarpal neck fracture is seen. A scaphoid fracture is now appreciated. Note absence of radioscaphoid arthritis. (**e**). Coronal CT shows distal third fracture with bone resorption. (**f**). Sagittal CT shows cystic change at fracture site with significant humpback deformity. (**g**). Intraoperative fluoroscopy showing radiolunate fixation. A transverse distal scaphoid large joystick wire was used to achieve reduction and then driven into the capitate to maintain alignment. Two wires stabilize a bicortical iliac crest bone graft. (**h**). 13 months after surgery and after wire removal at 10 weeks postop; PA radiograph shows scaphoid healing. (**i**). Pa ulnar deviation shows scaphoid and graft moves as a unit with healing. (**j**). Lateral shows maintenance of neutral radiolunate angle without DISI deformity. (**k**). Final wrist flexion. (**l**). Final wrist extension

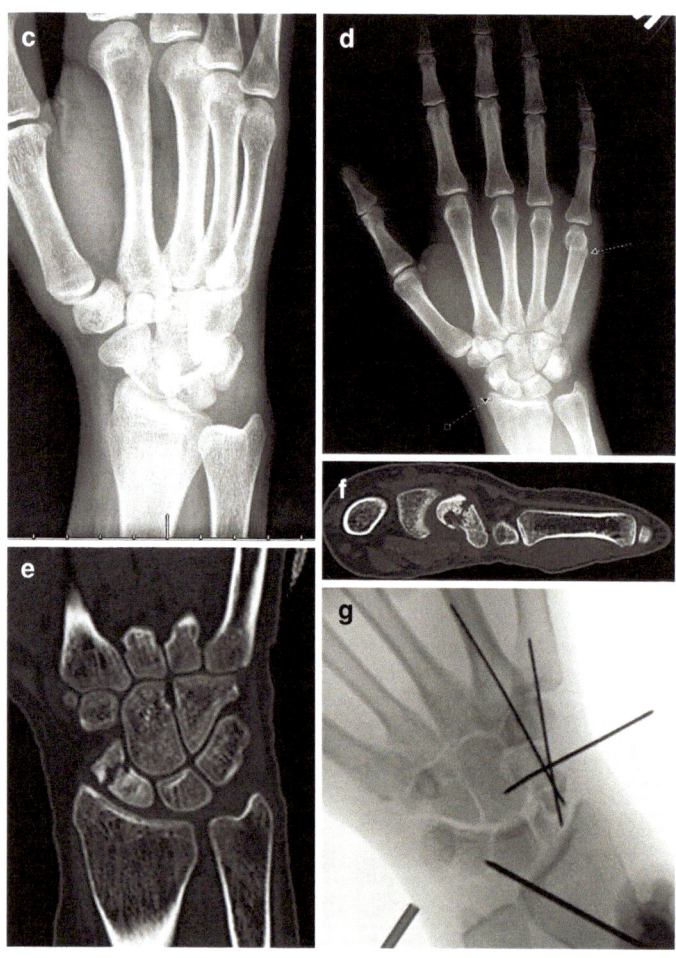

Figure 10.2 (continued)

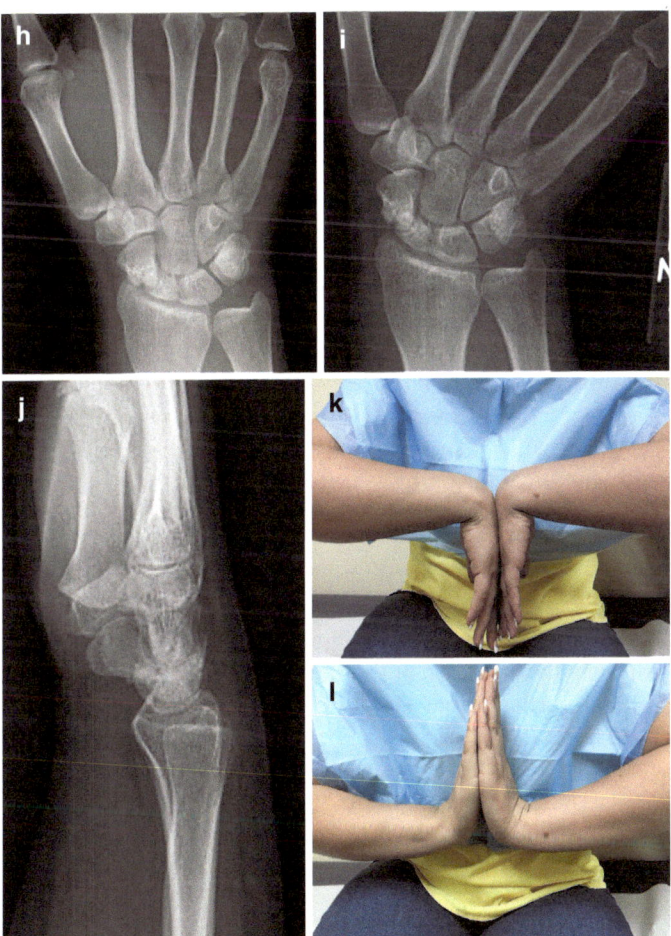

FIGURE 10.2 (continued)

Diagnostic Evaluation

Plain Radiographs

Plain radiographs remain the primary imaging modality and in most instances are sufficient to diagnose scaphoid fractures and determine treatment. The following neutral forearm rotation wrist radiographs should be obtained: extended finger PA, an ulnar deviated PA, and lateral (Figs. 10.1 and 10.2). A 15-degree pronated oblique is also obtained. Radiographs should be analyzed to determine scaphoid fracture line based on thirds as treatment varies based on proximal, middle (waist), or distal third location. Proximal pole sclerosis suggests avascular necrosis. Cystic changes within the scaphoid and lunate extension [dorsal intercalated segment instability (DISI)] as evidence by increased scapholunate and radiolunate angles suggest a fracture in which intrascaphoid angulation is present (humpback deformity). Intercarpal joint widening or step-offs (disruption of Gilula's arc) suggest an associated ligamentous injury. Joint space narrowing and osteophyte formation at the radial styloid-scaphoid and capitolunate articulations should be noted as they may indicate need for salvage reconstruction may include proximal row carpectomy or scaphoidectomy with 4-corner arthrodesis rather than fracture fixation.

If initial radiographs are normal but there is a high index of suspicion for a scaphoid fracture; either immobilize the wrist in a short arm thumb spica cast and repeat radiographs in 2–3 weeks, or consider advanced imaging.

MRI

If initial radiographs are normal, but the radial wrist pain and need for immobilization precludes the ability of the patient to work, and several weeks' delay in diagnosis would create financial or family challenges, MRI can be performed. In most cases, a non-contrast closed MRI from a facility with a 1.5 T or greater field strength, using a dedicated wrist coil, is the preferred study technique. If there is a substantial likelihood for

an associated ligament injury, a MR arthrogram with intraarticular gadolinium will increase the sensitivity of detecting a
ligamentous injury. This is particularly helpful in chronic
scaphoid non-unions, where a decision for fracture repair versus a salvage procedure would be indicated. If there is a need
to assess scaphoid vascularity, such as in a chronic proximal
pole fracture, a pre- and post-intravenous contrast MRI is the
optimal study to perform. A low-intensity signal within the
proximal pole on T1 and T2 images with failure to enhance
postcontrast administration indicates avascular necrosis.

CT Scan

A CT scan with axial images acquired in the plane of the long
axis of the scaphoid including sagittal and coronal reconstruc-
tions can be useful to obtain in an occult suspected fracture
(Figs. 10.1c–e and 10.2e, f). However, CT may be preferred
over MRI in most scaphoid waist or distal non-unions with low
risk for avascular necrosis to assess amount of bone loss, fracture angulation, and capitolunate angulation.

Treatment

Treatment is often dependent on fracture location, time from
injury, associated injuries, and type of work/activities, and
smoking status. No consensus exists on optimal type of hardware, surgical approach, or type of bone graft [1].

Non-displaced Distal Third/Waist Fractures

These are predominantly treated with non-operative immobilization in a well-molded thumb spica short arm cast with the
thumb IP joint freely mobile. Casting ensures patient compli-
ance with recommended full-time immobilization. However,
in a highly reliable patient or one who refuses casting, a
removable custom or prefabricated orthoses could be considered. Patients typically follow up at 2–3 weeks intervals for

cast changes and radiographs until union around 8–10 weeks. If healing is suggested, they are placed into a removable orthosis and started with gentle rehabilitation.

Displaced Scaphoid Waist/Proximal Pole Fractures

Acute proximal pole fractures are treated with an open dorsal approach to accurately align the fracture and place antegrade internal fixation with K wires or small headless compression screws depending on fragment size and fracture stability. Chronic proximal pole non-unions require additional pre- and intraoperative assessments of vascularity to determine if non- or vascularized bone graft is feasible or whether to undergo salvage treatment. Operative fixation of displaced scaphoid waist fractures can occur through either a dorsal or palmar approach [2]. Some surgeons prefer to use arthroscopic assistance to view the fracture and ensure there is no articular cartilage step-off, which is facilitated by a dorsal approach. The dorsal approach is typically through the interval between the third and fourth compartments with capsular dissection stopping proximal to the dorsal ridge in order to prevent injury to the tenuous dorsal blood supply. Reduction maneuvers and supplemental temporary fixation techniques are applicable to both surgical approaches.

Surgical Technique: Volar Approach

The patient is positioned supine with the arm extended on a radiolucent hand table. After exsanguination and tourniquet inflation, a volar-modified Bruner incision is made over the palmar radial wrist centered over the flexor carpi radialis (FCR) tendon. The FCR sheath is opened and the tendon is retracted ulnarly. The palmar capsule is opened to expose the scaphoid. Initially it may be difficult to identify the fracture site as the proximal half of the scaphoid is covered by the volar rim of the radius. If the fracture is well-aligned and does not angulate with wrist passive motion, the stable cartilage shell is left intact and fixation is placed.

If the scaphoid is displaced, unstable, impacted with intrascaphoid angulation, has cystic bone loss, or wrist extension creates malalignment precluding optimal guide wire placement, temporary intercarpal or radiocarpal fixation should be considered. When the scapholunate ligament is intact and the proximal pole fragment is mobile, the proximal scaphoid will follow the lunate. Thus, on lateral imaging if lunate extension is present, the wrist should be flexed until a neutral radiolunate angle is obtained [3]. A percutaneous antegrade radiolunate K wire is placed with a starting point in the fourth compartment in an adult (Fig. 10.1f) or the second compartment in a skeletally immature patient (Fig. 10.3). This obtains and stabilizes the proximal scaphoid in the correct anatomic position. The radiolunate wire is cut and bent outside skin and rotated so it lays flat on the wrist. Folded towels should

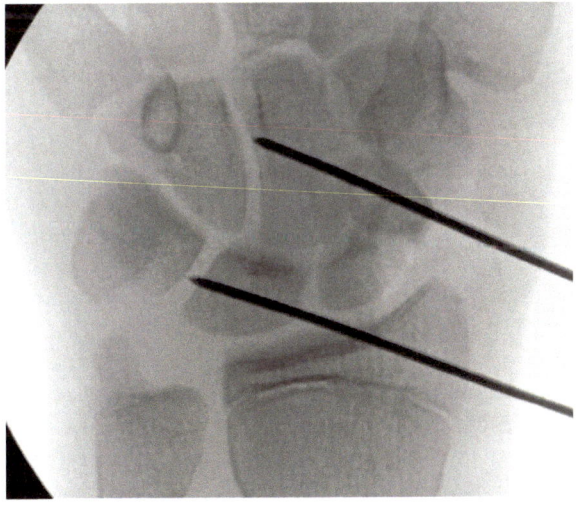

FIGURE 10.3 Skeletally immature patient with scaphoid waist fracture with radial styloid-lunate transarticular wire placed through second compartment to avoid transphyseal placement. A distal scaphocapitate wire stabilizes the distal pole

be placed on the hand table to help prevent the wire from inadvertently cutting the drapes. Extending the wrist into a neutral or mildly extended position should then align the midcarpal joint with the distal scaphoid extending to follow the capitate. This corrects the scaphoid angulation and DISI deformity. If the distal pole does not extend, a joystick K wire can be placed in the distal pole and manipulated to extend the distal scaphoid and then driven into the capitate or trapezium to maintain the corrected position (Fig. 10.2g). An antirotation wire is placed off of the central axis to stabilize the fracture (Figs. 10.1g and 10.2g). The nonparallel antirotation guide wire should be placed sufficiently far from the centered guide wire so it does not bind during drilling or screw placement. The central axis guide wire is placed either through the trapezium or by making a small arthrotomy in the scaphotrapezial joint and hyperextending the metacarpal to expose the distal scaphoid pole [4].The measurement guide is placed over the central guide wire. The author prefers to subtract at least 6 mm to obtain the screw length, which should be 20–24 mm in most patients. This permits the screw to be seated fully within bone, accounts for fracture compression, and permits measurement error with transtrapzeial placement where the trapezium and joint space distances need to be estimated and also subtracted when the measurement guide is placed over the guidewire. An alternative is to start drilling through the trapezium up to the distal pole of the scaphoid and then stop. The depth gauge is then placed through the drill hole to better estimate wire and screw length. The wire is then advanced through the proximal scaphoid and possibly into the distal radius to prevent wire removal if binding occurs during drilling. The cannulated conical drill is used through the trapezium if not previously drilled and into the scaphoid upto the proximal pole subchondral bone. The screw driver is dipped in saline or a small amount of bone wax is applied to prevent the screwdriver shaft tip from binding excessively to the screw head. Once the screw is advanced where several threads have crossed the fracture site to engage the proximal fragment, the antirota-

tion wire is removed to permit compression. Manual stabilization of the distal fragment by grasping the metacarpal base/
trapezium and applying an axial load can help prevent fragment rotation. The guide wires are removed. The wrist should
be passively ranged under live fluoroscopy to confirm fracture stability and ensure there is sufficient motion in all
planes to indicate the scaphoid is appropriately aligned.
Multiple PA, AP, lateral, pronated, and supinated oblique
images should be obtained to assess screw length [5]. If a
screw length is too long, it is the author's preference to leave
it prominent at the scaphotrapezial joint rather than the
radioscaphoid joint. The scaphotrapezial joint appears to be
more forgiving than the radioscaphoid joint and late screw
removal has not been necessary due distal screw prominence.
The capsule is closed with absorbable braided 2–0 or 3–0
suture and a thumb spica splint applied.

Bone Graft

For most scaphoid waist nonunions, nonvascularized cancellous bone from the metaphyseal portion of the distal radius is
used, often approaching the radial styloid through the second
compartment through a separate dorsal incision [6, 7]. This
places the donor site within the same extremity, makes
postop wound care easier, and is better tolerated as the pain
is in the same region. After fracture site preparation and provisional reduction is achieved, bone wax can be packed into
the scaphoid nonunion site to create a mold of the bone void
(personal communication Kagan Ozer, MD). The wax is then
removed and measured with a ruler to determine dimensions
and shape of the required bone graft. Using a ¼ inch straight
osteotome, three sides of a rectangle are cut radial to Lister's
tubercle with the distal cut made first 1.5–2 cm proximal to
the articular surface. Then a curved osteotome is used to lever
up the cortical trapdoor hinging open the cortex on the uncut
fourth side, leaving the periosteum and a portion of bone
intact. Cancellous bone is removed with straight and curved

curettes. The donor site may or may not be filled with bone graft substitute. The trapdoor is closed and the periosteum is repaired with 3–0 or 4–0 suture. If structural graft is needed a larger block of corticocancellous bone can be harvested without formation of the trapdoor.

The curetted cancellous bone fragments are placed into a 5-cc syringe and gentle compression is performed [7]. Blood that is expressed from the syringe tip is collected in a small specimen cup or lid. A K wire is placed through the syringe tip to gently back the graft out. The graft is soaked in the extruded blood to retrieve bone marrow cells. The graft can be placed either before or after central and anti-rotation guide wires.

Iliac crest may be utilized when severe humpback deformity with larger volumetric and cortical bone loss exists, in proximal pole non-unions where a higher density of osteoprogenitor stem cells and osteoblasts are desired, or with open distal radial growth plates where harvest could cause a growth arrest. Similar to the description above, cancellous only bone may be harvested through a trapdoor window, or a bi- or tricortical graft may be harvested using a bone wax mold to assist in graft size and shape determination. It is not always necessary to use a compression screw with bone graft. When stability is achieved with wires alone and good graft impaction and stability can be achieved around the wires, lack of screw placement may leave a larger amount of bone surface available for healing. However, staged wire removal will be needed after fracture union (Fig. 10.2). Multiple additional vascularized graft options exist with indications and outcomes for different graft types summarized by other authors [8].

References

1. Pinder RM, Brkljac M, Rix L, Muir L, Brewster M. Treatment of scaphoid nonunion: a systematic review of the existing evidence. J Hand Surg [Am]. 2015;40(9):1797–1805.e3.

2. Jeon I, Micic ID, Oh C, Park B, Kim P. Percutaneous screw fixation for scaphoid fracture: a comparison between the dorsal and the volar approaches. J Hand Surg [Am]. 2009;34(2):228–36.e1.

3. Tomaino M, King J, Pizillo M. Correction of lunate malalignment when bone grafting scaphoid nonunion with humpback deformity: rationale and results of a technique revisited. J Hand Surg [Am]. 2000;25(2):322–9.

4. Meermans G, Verstreken F. A comparison of 2 methods for scaphoid central screw placement from a volar approach. J Hand Surg [Am]. 2011;36(10):1669–74.

5. Kim RY, Lijtten EC, Strauch RJ. Pronated oblique view in assessing proximal scaphoid articular cannulated screw penetration. J Hand Surg [Am]. 2008;33A:1274–7.

6. Sayegh ET, Strauch RJ. Graft choice in the management of unstable scaphoid nonunion: a systematic review. J Hand Surg [Am]. 2014;39(8):1500–6.

7. Cohen MS, Jupiter JB, Fallahi K, Shukla SK. Scaphoid waist nonunion with humpback deformity treated without structural bone graft. J Hand Surg [Am]. 2013;38A:701–5.

8. Jones Jr DB, Rhee PC, Shin AY. Vascularized bone grafts for scaphoid nonunions. J Hand Surg [Am]. 2012;40(9):1791–6.

Chapter 11
Lunate and Perilunate Dislocations: Tips and Tricks for Problem Fractures

Angela A. Wang and Brittany Garcia

Background

Lunate and perilunate injuries result from high-energy traumatic insult to the carpus. Typical injury mechanisms include motor vehicle accidents and falls (most often from a significant height). Perilunate injuries should be thought of as a spectrum of injury ranging from purely ligamentous disruption to fractures and dislocations of the carpal bones. With increasing injury severity comes progressive instability of the wrist. Mayfield et al. described and classified the patterns of perilunar injury and resultant carpal instability (Table 11.1) [1]. They determined the most common mechanism of injury is caused by a force applied through the extended, ulnarly deviated wrist with concurrent intercarpal supination [1, 2]. These forces result in the more common dorsal perilunate dislocation.

A. A. Wang (✉) · B. Garcia
Department of Orthopaedic Surgery, University of Utah, Salt Lake City, UT, USA
e-mail: angela.wang@hsc.utah.edu

© Springer Nature Switzerland AG 2020
D. S. Horwitz et al. (eds.), *Tips and Tricks for Problem Fractures, Volume I*,
https://doi.org/10.1007/978-3-030-38274-2_11

TABLE 11.1 Ligamentous disruption and Mayfield stage

Ligamentous disruption and Mayfield stage			
Stage I	Scapholunate dissociation		
Stage II	Scapholunate + dissociation	Lunocapitate compromise	
Stage III	Scapholunate + dissociation	Lunocapitate + compromise	Lunotriquetral compromise
Stage IV	Scapholunate + dissociation	Lunocapitate + compromise	Lunotriquetral + compromise	Lunate rotates/ dislocates

Diagnosis

Despite the severity of these injuries, carpal dislocations are frequently missed. A thorough history, physical exam, and quality imaging are necessary for accurate diagnosis. Exam findings are dependent on chronicity and severity of injury. Acute injuries can present with pain, wrist swelling, median nerve paresthesias, and capitate prominence dorsally. Chronic or missed injuries may be less obvious.

Radiographs are the most beneficial initial diagnostic imaging modality. To adequately evaluate for perilunate and lunate injuries, initial radiographic imaging should include posteroanterior (PA), lateral, scaphoid, and 45-degree semi-pronated oblique wrist views [3]. PA radiographs provide important information regarding normal carpal alignment, carpal fractures, and associated radial styloid fractures. Gilula's lines and the lesser and greater arcs help define normal carpal relationships on PA wrist radiographs (Figs. 11.1 and 11.2) [2, 3]. Lateral radiographs

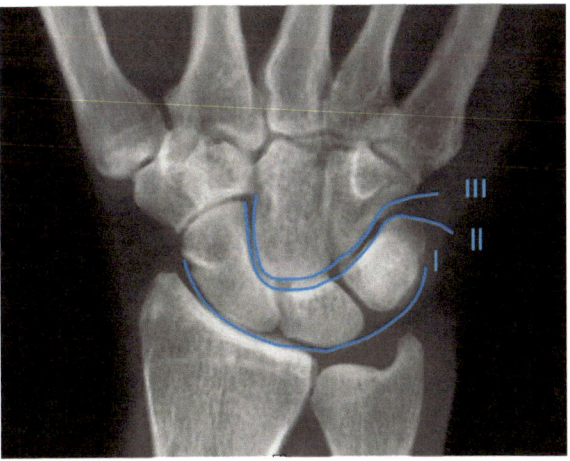

FIGURE 11.1 Normal carpal alignment on the PA view evaluated by Gilula's lines (I, II, III). A break or step-off in Gilula's lines indicates displacement of the normal intercarpal relationships [3]

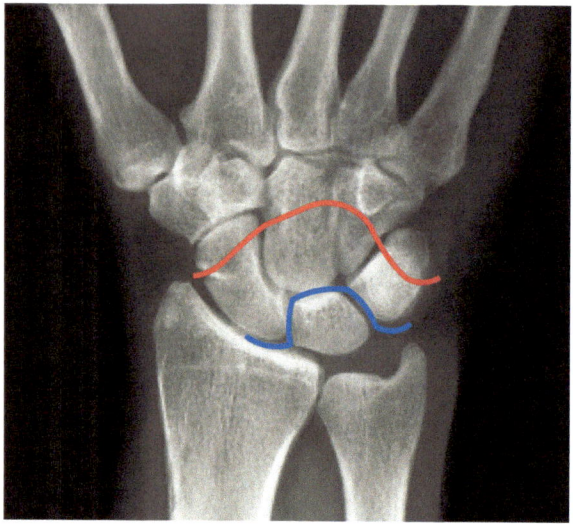

FIGURE 11.2 Lesser and greater arcs. Blue/lower line – lesser arc injury which indicates purely ligamentous injury pattern. Red/upper line – greater arc injury which indicates injury through both ligaments and carpal bones (e.g. trans-scaphoid perilunate dislocation)

are most helpful for closely scrutinizing the co-linearity of the radius, lunate, and capitate. The lateral radiograph is also very important for visualization of the more common dorsal perilunate dislocation, characterized by the capitate sitting dorsal to the lunate with maintenance of the lunate within the lunate fossa [1]. Oblique wrist radiographs may be helpful for further characterization of injury pattern and identification of subtle fractures not well visualized on other images [3].

Formal postreduction radiographs are important and may show previously missed subtle carpal fractures, including fractures of the scaphoid, radial styloid, capitate, and trique-trum. An ulnar deviation or scaphoid magnification view after successful reduction is helpful for identifying or clarify-ing scaphoid fractures that may not have been noted on initial imaging. Computed tomography (CT) and magnetic resonance imaging (MRI) following initial reduction may not be indicated but can assist with evaluation for occult fractures, ligamentous injury, and details of fracture fragments [2]. Inadequate or poor imaging is a frequent reason for missed injury.

Classification

The Mayfield Classification is frequently used to describe perilunate injuries and is based on a cadaveric study performed by Mayfield et al. in 1980 [1].

Lunate dislocations are different from perilunate dislocations. Perilunate dislocations are characterized by dorsal dislocation of the carpus with retention of the lunate within the lunate fossa of the distal radius (Fig. 11.3a). Lunate dislocations are defined by dislocation of the lunate bone from its

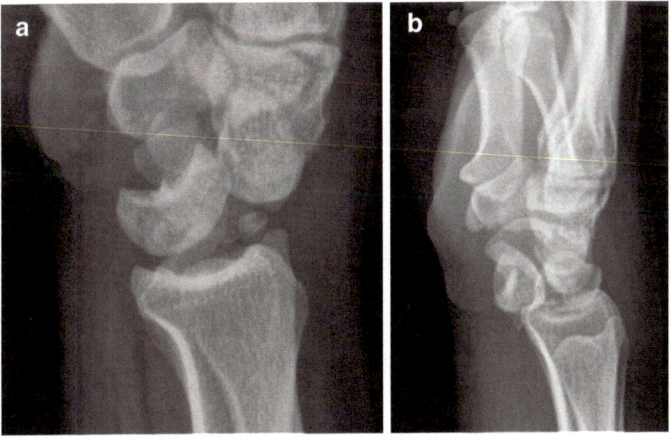

FIGURE 11.3 (**a**). Stage III perilunate dislocation with maintenance of the lunate in the lunate fossa. (**b**). Stage IV perilunate dislocation. Patient was irreducible in the emergency department. "Spilled tea cup sign" – lunate tipped over volarly

TABLE 11.2 Common radiographic findings associated with stage of injury

Common radiographic findings associated with stage of injury	
Stage I	Scapholunate interval widening
Stage II	Capitate subluxates or dislocates dorsally with respect to the lunate
Stage III	Lunotriquetral interval widening; avulsion fractures of the triquetrum; capitate dorsally dislocated
Stage IV	Lunate dislocates. Triangulated lunate (PA view, Fig. 11.4). Capitate may articulate with lunate fossa

anatomic position in the lunate fossa, leaving the proximal pole of the capitate to articulate in the lunate fossa (Fig. 11.3b). Most commonly the lunate will dislocate volarly (Table 11.2 and Fig. 11.4).

Closed Management

Management of perilunate injuries depends on injury pattern and severity. However, in the acute setting initial treatment should begin with an attempted closed reduction. Even with acceptable closed reduction, surgical stabilization of these injuries is favored due to persistent intercarpal instability from ligamentous injury [2]. If median nerve symptoms are present or there is concern for acute carpal tunnel syndrome, urgent reduction, either in the emergency department (ER) or the operating room, should be a priority [2]. If median nerve symptoms persist or worsen after closed reduction in the ER, then emergent surgical intervention is warranted [2, 4]. Even with a successful closed reduction, surgery should be scheduled in an urgent rather than leisurely fashion, particularly with a scaphoid fracture, which is often widely displaced in this type of injury (suggesting a significant disruption to the vascular supply).

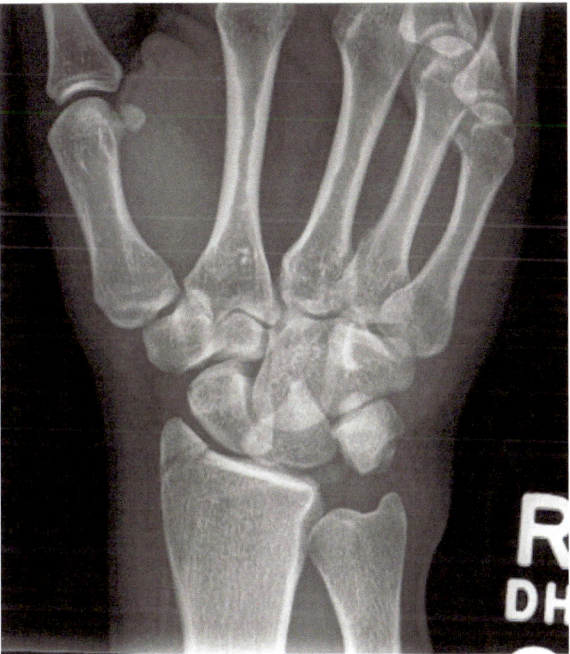

FIGURE 11.4 PA radiograph of a stage IV transradial styloid lunate dislocation showing overlapping of the capitate and lunate and the "triangle sign"

Closed Reduction

The purpose of immediate, gentle, closed reduction is to take pressure off the cartilage and important neurovascular structures. Closed reduction is most commonly performed in the emergency department. Both conscious sedation and local blocks (e.g. Bier block) can provide adequate analgesia for a successful reduction. It is helpful to begin by hanging the injured extremity in finger traction with the elbow flexed to 90 degrees to allow the soft tissues to relax and assist with a more successful reduction [2, 3]. Often times, reduction is easier than anticipated, owing to the significant disruption of ligamentous structures. Frequently the carpal bones are "loose" and can be reduced with gentle manipulation but may not always stay reduced after pressure and traction is removed.

Reduction Maneuver

- Place patient supine on the stretcher, lying flat
- Place hand in finger traction with the elbow flexed to 90 degrees and 5–15 pounds of counter traction hanging from the upper arm (approximately 5–15 minutes) [2–4].
- Direction of applied reduction force depends on injury pattern.
  - Dorsal dislocations (capitate dislocated dorsal to lunate) which are the most common, are reduced by extending the wrist, apply longitudinal traction with ulnar deviation, followed by radial deviation with palmar flexion of the wrist [1, 2, 4]. During this maneuver volar pressure should be applied to the lunate and dorsal pressure on the capitate to reduce the capitate while preventing the lunate from displacing [2, 4].

Splinting

After postreduction radiographs are completed and acceptable reduction is confirmed, the patient should be placed into a well-padded, volarly molded thumb spica splint with the wrist in a neutral position. As discussed previously, the patient may undergo surgery in an elective fashion but with emphasis on intervention sooner rather than later, particularly for trans-scaphoid fracture dislocations (expedited surgery will also avoid capsular scarring, which will make inter- and intracarpal reductions more difficult later).

Surgical Management

Surgical Indications

- Immediate: Acute carpal tunnel syndrome or persistent median nerve symptoms following closed reduction; failure to attain acceptable closed reduction; open injuries
- Elective/urgent: stabilization of ligamentous injury and/or fracture fixation to regain anatomic carpal alignment following acceptable closed reduction [2].

Approaches to the Wrist

Three main approaches are used to gain access to the carpus: dorsal, volar, and combined volar and dorsal. The approach used is largely surgeon dependent as well as contingent on the particular injury pattern and need for access to structures. Goals of surgical management include fracture fixation, ligamentous stabilization, and anatomic reduction with restoration of normal carpal alignment [2].

If the lunate has been dislocated and/or is irreducible or the patient has symptoms of acute carpal tunnel syndrome, begin with a volar approach. If not, you may begin with the more common dorsal approach which allows for access to the scapholunate (SL) ligament. This is done by making a longitudinal incision dorsally over the III and IV extensor compartments. The extensor tendons are identified, the retinaculum is opened, and the tendons are retracted radially (III) and ulnarly (IV). At this point the authors typically resect the terminal, sensory branch of the PIN running on the floor of the fourth compartment. The capsule is then opened by making a radially based, V-shaped ligament sparing capsular flap which allows for a secure, more anatomic repair at the end of the case (Fig. 11.5). The carpal bones are inspected for cartilage damage, ligament disruption, and any loose fragments are removed. SL ligament disruption and scaphoid

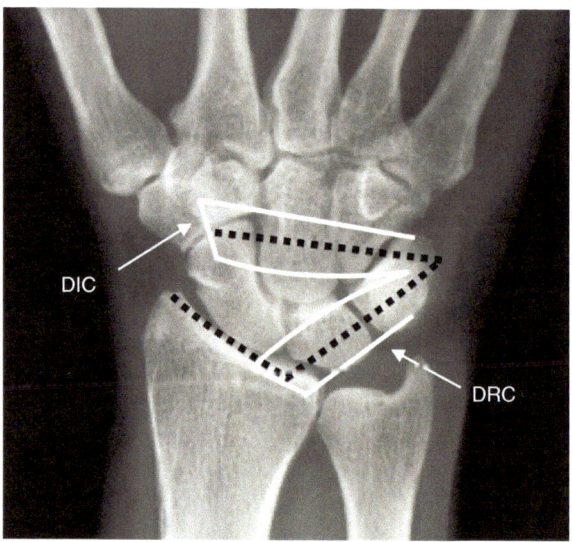

FIGURE 11.5 V-shaped, ligament splitting capsular incision to make a flap along the distal intercarpal ligament (DIC) and the dorsal radoiocarpal ligament (DRC). Ligaments indicated in white, dashed line denote longitudinal capsular incision which is then reflected radially

fractures are then easily visualized. Upon inspection, it is not uncommon to see injury to the head of the capitate as well, which portends a poorer outcome. Rarely, patients will have both a ligament disruption and a fracture; usually, it is either one or the other.

If there is a scaphoid fracture, it should be fixed first. Sturdy Kirschner wires (K-wires) are placed into each scaphoid fracture fragment to aid in reduction (at least 0.54 mm), followed by fixation of choice (the authors favor a headless compressive screw) (Fig. 11.6a). If there is no fracture, the K-wires are still placed in the scaphoid and the lunate to aid in the reduction of these bones. With the reduction held, two K-wires are then placed from the scaphoid into the lunate and the reduction/pin placement is verified on the Mini

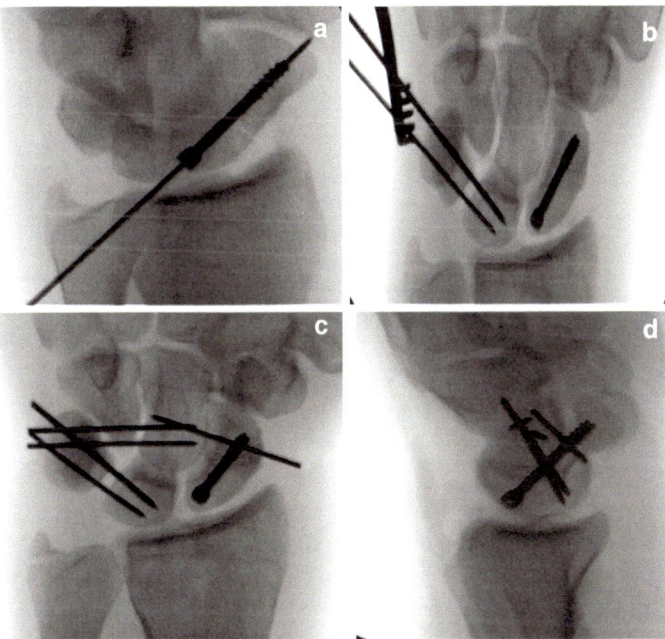

FIGURE 11.6 (**a**–**d**) Sequential fixation beginning with the scaphoid (**a**), followed by fixation of the lunotriquetral interval (**b**), and lastly triquetrum-hamate-capitate fixation (**c**, **d**)

C-arm. The SL ligament is then identified and repaired; in our experience it is usually avulsed off the lunate. It may be fixed using bone tunnels or suture anchors (our preference) and a braided non-absorbable suture (Fig. 11.7). The SL angle should be restored to 45–60 degrees, and the capitolunate angle should be restored to 0–15 degrees on intraoperative imaging.

Next, K-wires are placed across the lunotriquetral joint (Fig. 11.6b). A pointed reduction forceps may be used to gently squeeze the two carpal bones together if they are widely separated. Two K-wires provide better rotational stability than one, but it can sometimes be difficult to place the second wire given the limited "real estate" in the lunate. If a

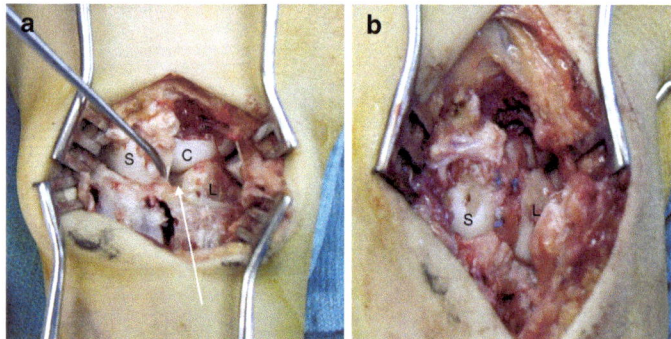

FIGURE 11.7 (**a**). Showing SL diastasis. (**b**). Suture repair of the SL ligament. S scaphoid, L lunate, C capitate. White arrow points to scapholunate diastasis

scaphoid fracture has been fixed, and the SL ligament is intact, it may not be necessary to place a scaphocapitate (SC) pin. If not, a SC K-wire should be placed to protect and take force off the SL repair. One to two triquetrum-hamate-capitate (THC) pins may also be placed for anatomic reduction; the dorsal capsule is repaired, followed by the retinaculum (extensor pollicis longus can be left outside the retinaculum if desired).

The volar approach is necessary if there are carpal tunnel symptoms, or if the lunate is irreducible. In these cases, the lunate has usually herniated through the volar capsule. A longitudinal carpal tunnel-type incision is made in line with the fourth ray in the palm. It is zig-zagged slightly to cross the transverse wrist crease proximally (Fig. 11.8). The palmar fascia is then divided followed by release of the transverse carpal ligament. Here, the lunate may be encountered and reduced back through the volar capsule (followed by fixation via dorsal approach as above). After retracting the median nerve and tendons aside, a significant tear in the floor of the carpal canal/volar capsule can often be appreciated. While the necessity of repair of this structure is not clear, it can be satisfying to place a few sutures to repair this rent. Literature

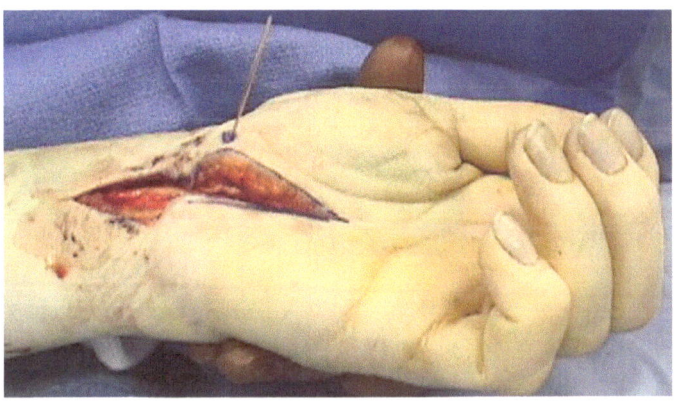

FIGURE 11.8 Extended carpal tunnel incision for a volar approach to the carpal tunnel and carpus in a patient with an irreducible lunate dislocation

is mixed regarding the need for a volar approach, and the only clear indications are carpal tunnel symptoms and an irreducible lunate.

K-wires used for fixation may be left outside or cut just beneath the skin. The authors prefer the latter, as we strive for leaving the pins in place at least 9 weeks or even longer if tolerated by the skin and soft tissues. The patient is immobilized in the volar thumb spica splint for 1–2 weeks, followed by a cast for 6–8 weeks.

A proximal row carpectomy or wrist fusion may be indicated during acute injury in the setting of advanced age or significant pre-existing arthritis, acute-catastrophic cartilage damage, or if patients are sick and high risk for prolonged or repeat general anesthesia.

Management of Chronic Perilunar Injuries

Management of chronic perilunar injuries can be more complex. If open reduction with internal fixation is not appropriate given the length of time from injury, alternative surgical options are necessary. Proximal row carpectomy is considered a reasonable salvage procedure for chronic perilunar injuries. For advanced midcarpal and radiocarpal arthritis, partial or total wrist arthrodesis may be indicated [4].

Complications and Outcomes

Prognosis depends on timely recognition and treatment of lunate and perilunate injuries as well as adequacy of reduction and fixation. The most common complications associated with perilunar injuries are missed or inaccurate diagnosis, median nerve dysfunction, pin tract infections, symptomatic hardware, carpal malunion or nonunion, chronic instability, and post-traumatic arthritis [1, 2, 4]. Following management of perilunar injuries, long-term outcomes show loss of motion, pain, and diminished grip strength as common symptoms. Midcarpal and radial carpal arthroses on radiographs are common; however, it does not necessarily correlate well with functional outcomes.

The patient should be informed at the time of surgery as to the gravity of injury, possible need for additional surgery, and the high likelihood of sequelae. These injuries are technically challenging to fix as a well as biologically tricky (blood supply to the scaphoid as well as carpal ligaments is scarce), but prompt attention and restoration of the carpal alignment affords the best chance at achieving a good outcome.

References

1. Mayfield JK, Johnson RP, Kilcoyne RK. Carpal dislocations: pathomechanics and progressive perilunar instability. J Hand Surg Am. 1980;5(3):226–41.
2. Stanbury SJ, Elfar JC. Perilunate dislocation and perilunate fracture-dislocation. J Am Acad Orthop Surg. 2011;19(9):554–62.

3. Wolfe S, Pederson W, Hotchkiss R, Kozin S. Greens operative hand surgery. 6th ed. New York: Elsevier; 2010. Carpal instability Chapter 15.
4. Kozin SH. Perilunate injuries: diagnosis and treatment. J Am Acad Orthop Surg. 1998;6(2):114–20.

Chapter 12
Metacarpal Fractures: Tips and Tricks

Anil Akoon and Joel Christian Klena

Metacarpal fractures account for up to 18% of all upper extremity fractures seen below the elbow [1]. The small finger sustains the most fractures followed by the ring, long, thumb, and index fingers [2]. Stable metacarpal fractures are traditionally treated with immobilization. There is no consensus on how to treat unstable metacarpal fractures. Ideally the fixation utilized should be stable enough to allow for early mobility to reduce the risk of stiffness [3]. Several cases are presented highlighting some of the many treatment methods available, each with their own advantages and disadvantages.

A. Akoon (✉)
Department of Orthopaedic Surgery, Geisinger Health System, Danville, PA, USA

J. C. Klena
Division of Hand Surgery, Department of Orthopaedic Surgery, Geisinger Medical Center, Danville, PA, USA

© Springer Nature Switzerland AG 2020
D. S. Horwitz et al. (eds.), *Tips and Tricks for Problem Fractures, Volume I*,
https://doi.org/10.1007/978-3-030-38274-2_12

Case 1: Closed Reduction Percutaneous Pinning

History

A 55-year-old right-hand-dominant male involved in an MVA sustained a closed, left, spiral oblique, small finger metacarpal shaft fracture (Fig. 12.1).

Indications

Maintenance of displaced spiral oblique fractures of the metacarpals via closed means is difficult. Operative treatment options include closed reduction and percutaneous pinning (CRPP), open reduction with lag screw or pin fixation, and open reduction with plate fixation. CRPP is the preferred method when the fracture is reducible using closed means. By preventing surgical dissection, the risk of adhesions and stiffness is reduced. Hardware irritation is minimized as pins are routinely removed at three to 4 weeks post-op. CRPP does introduce the potential risk for pin site irritation and, less commonly, infection [4].

Description of Operation

Under general LMA anesthesia, the patient was placed supine and the extremity placed on a hand table. A non-sterile tourniquet in the axilla was utilized. Under multiplanar fluoroscopic imaging, longitudinal traction was applied, and a pointed reduction clamp placed percutaneously to provide reduction. Two 0.045 K-wires were placed distally, each achieving bi-cortical fixation into both the small and ring finger metacarpals. The proximal pin was similarly placed across both metacarpals. The pins were cut and bent, and final images were obtained confirming reduction of the fracture site and pin placement (Fig. 12.2).

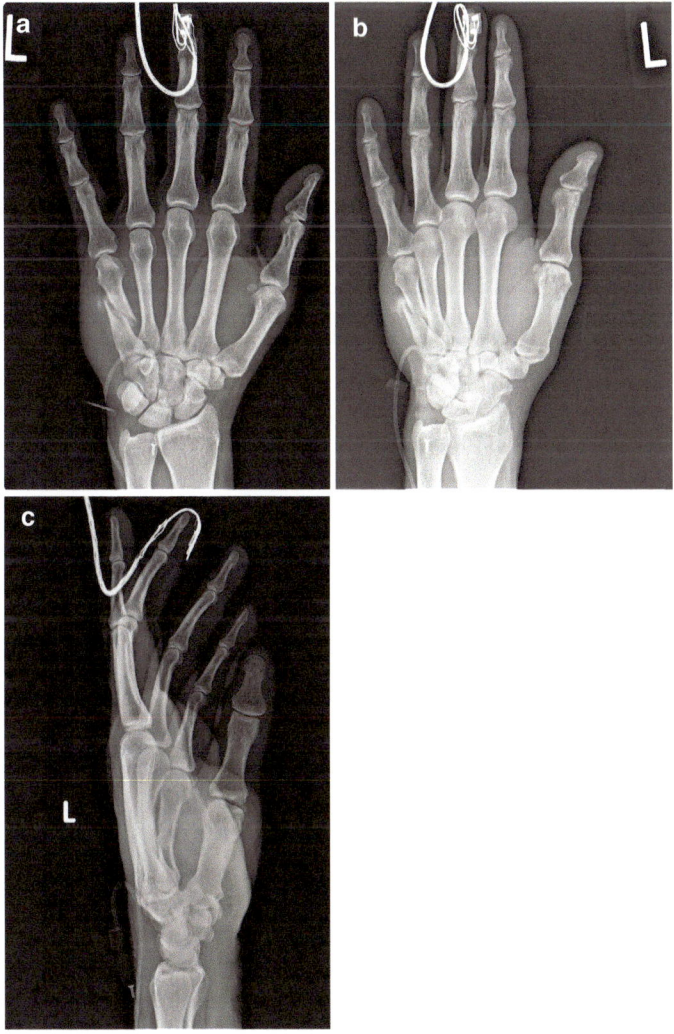

FIGURE 12.1 (**a–c**) Three x-ray views of a closed, left, spiral oblique, small finger metacarpal shaft fracture

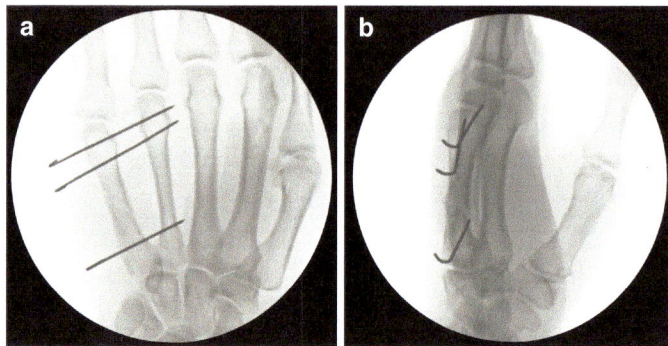

FIGURE 12.2 Intraoperative final fluoroscopy PA (**a**) and lateral (**b**) views of a closed, left, spiral oblique, small finger metacarpal fracture status post closed reduction and pinning

Post-Operative Course

An ulnar gutter cast was placed with follow-up at 10 days post-op for pin site check and fabrication of a custom thermoplast splint with occupational therapy. The pins were removed in clinic at 4 weeks post-op.

Case 2: Intramedullary Pin Fixation

History

A 44-year-old right-hand-dominant male status post a gunshot wound presented with an open, left metacarpal fracture of the ring finger with segmental bone loss (Fig. 12.3).

The injury underwent debridement and irrigation in the operating room with provisional fixation via two 0.062 K-wires placed to maintain length and gross alignment (Fig. 12.4).

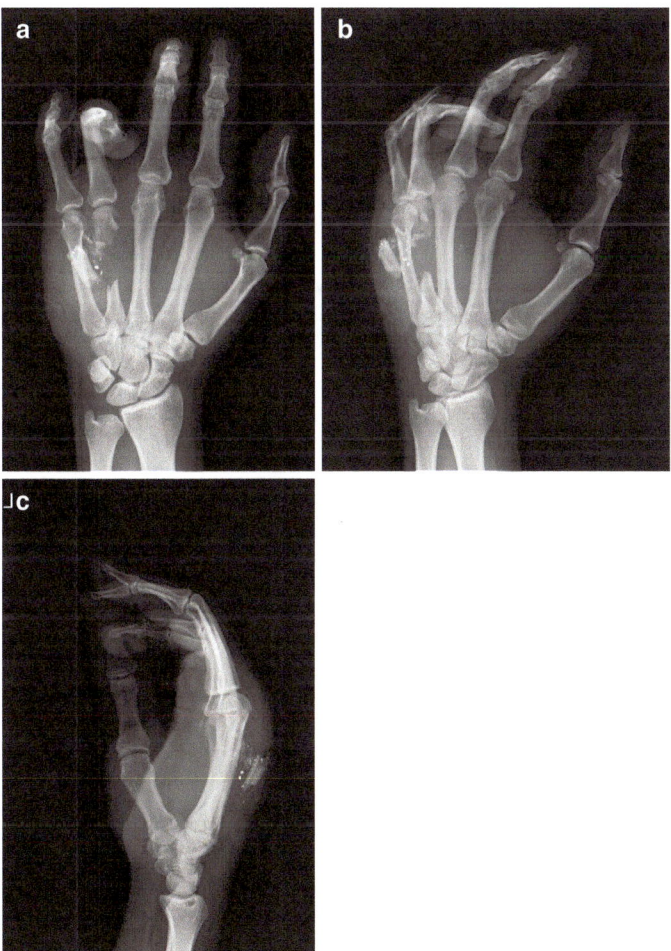

FIGURE 12.3 (**a–c**) Three x-ray views of an open, left, ring finger metacarpal fracture with segmental bone loss status post gunshot wound

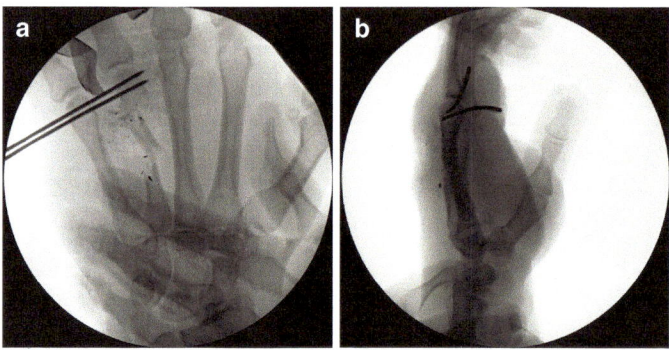

FIGURE 12.4 Intraoperative fluoroscopy PA (**a**) and lateral (**b**) views of a left ring finger metacarpal fracture provisionally pinned with two 0.062 K-wires

Indications

The patient had an open fracture with segmental loss of bone. Options for fracture stabilization include open reduction and percutaneous pinning, intramedullary (IM) fixation, bridge plating, or the use of an external fixator. Both structural and nonstructural autograft or allograft have been utilized to fill bone defects. The distal extension of the fracture made the use of pins preferential to plating with pins also minimizing additional soft tissue dissection.

Description of Operation

The dorsal exit wound was debrided with care taken to protect any remaining bone fragments and their soft tissue attachments. An intramedullary 0.062 K-wire was utilized to provide gross restoration of length and alignment. The wire was passed first through the segmental bone fragment, next into the proximal metacarpal shaft, and then shot-gunned into the distal fragment. Additional wires were then placed through the index metacarpal into the adjacent metacarpals.

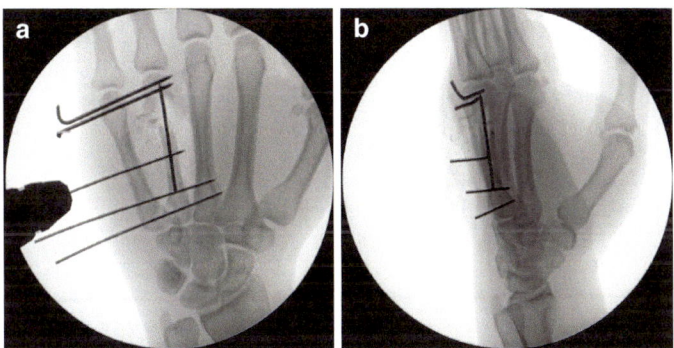

FIGURE 12.5 Intraoperative final fluoroscopy PA (**a**) and lateral (**b**) views of a left ring finger metacarpal fracture status post intramedullary pinning, parallel pinning to the adjacent digits and bone grafting

Cortico-cancellous bone graft was harvested from the dorsal distal radius with the bone graft placed into the defect (Fig. 12.5).

Post-operative Course

At 2 weeks post-op the patient was placed in a custom molded splint and motion initiated at the PIP and DIP joints. The pins remained until 2 months post-op with the IM pin permanently implanted. The patient achieved union (Fig.12.6).

Case 3: Low Profile Plate Fixation

History

A 20-year-old right-hand-dominant male football player sustained a closed, spiral oblique fracture of the left ring metacarpal (Fig. 12.7).

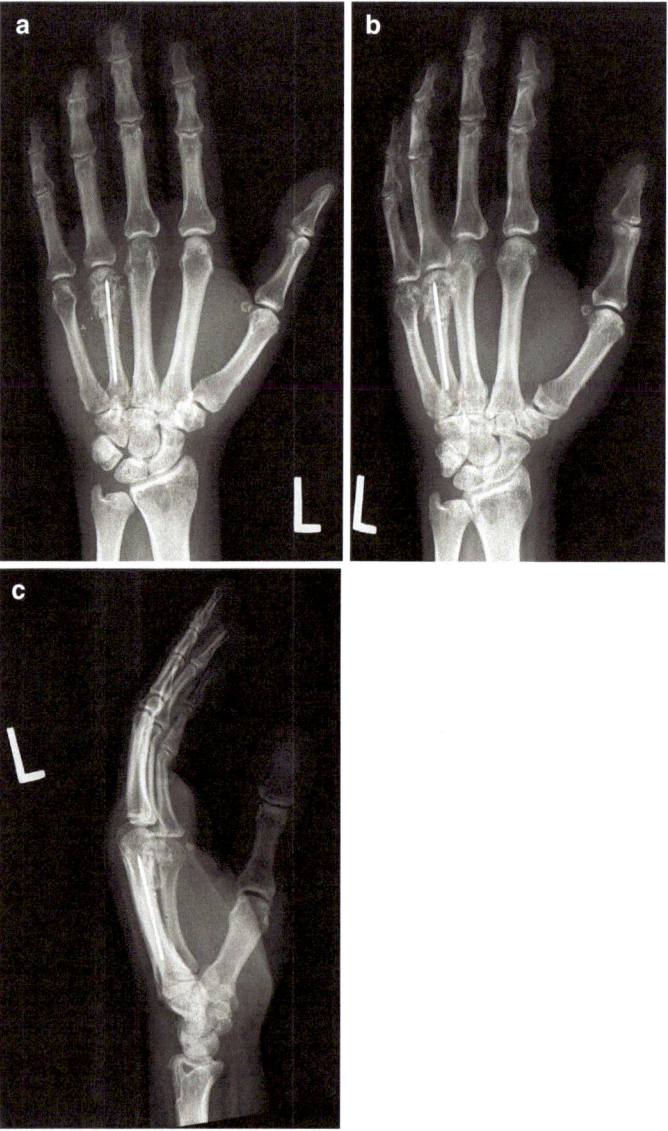

FIGURE 12.6 (**a–c**) Three x-ray views of an open, left, ring finger metacarpal fracture with segmental bone loss status post gunshot wound that has achieved union status post removal of provisional K-wires

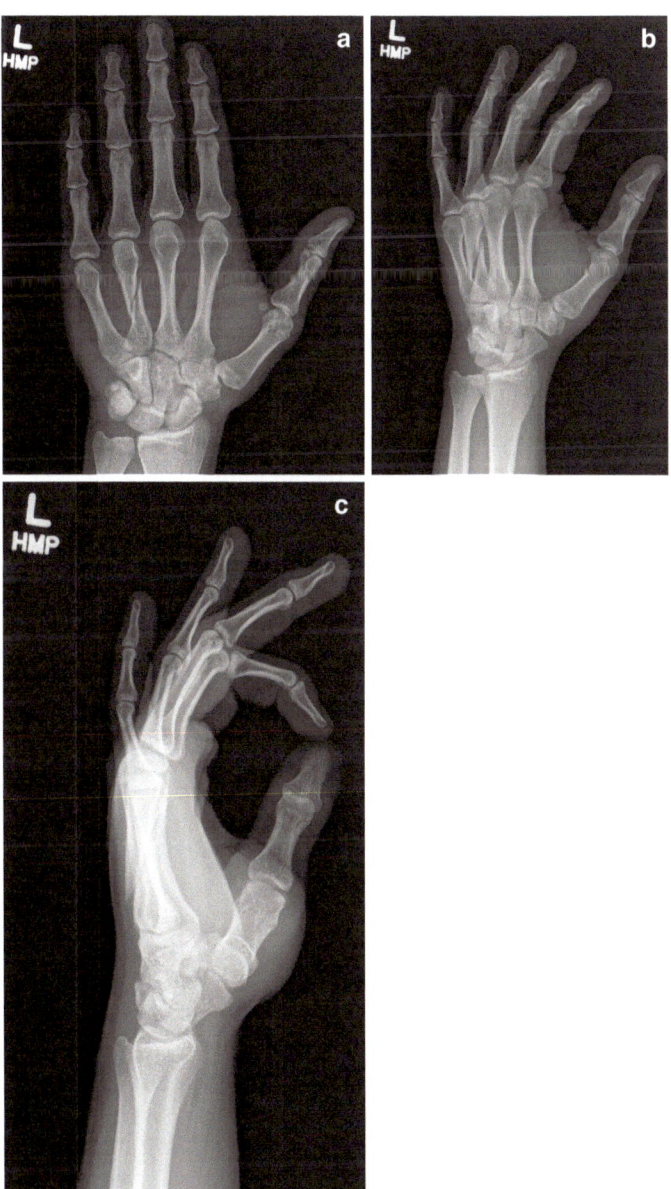

FIGURE 12.7 (**a–c**) Three x-ray views of a closed, spiral oblique fracture of the left ring metacarpal

Indications

With both shortening and malrotation, the fracture meets operative criteria. To allow an earlier return to play, open reduction was planned. The short segment of the oblique fracture renders lag screw fixation alone insufficient: open reduction and internal fixation with a low-profile plate was decided upon.

Description of Operation

A dorsal incision was made slightly ulnar to the metacarpal. The fracture was exposed and provisionally held with a K-wire with reduction verified under multi-planar imaging. A 1.5 mm T-plate was secured proximally and distally; centrally lag screws were placed through the plate (Fig. 12.8). The contrast between the lower profile plate is seen in comparison to a conventional plate (Fig. 12.9).

Post-operative Course

The patient returned on post-op day seven for a custom splint to initiate motion. Sutures were removed on post op day 14. At 3 weeks post-op the patient returned to play and casted for an additional 3 weeks before playing unprotected.

Case 4: Lag Screw/Plate Fixation

History

A 78-year-old right-hand-dominant male status post motor vehicle crash presented with closed, long oblique, spiral fractures of his right index, long, and ring metacarpals (Fig. 12.10). Concomitant pelvic and abdominal injuries were sustained.

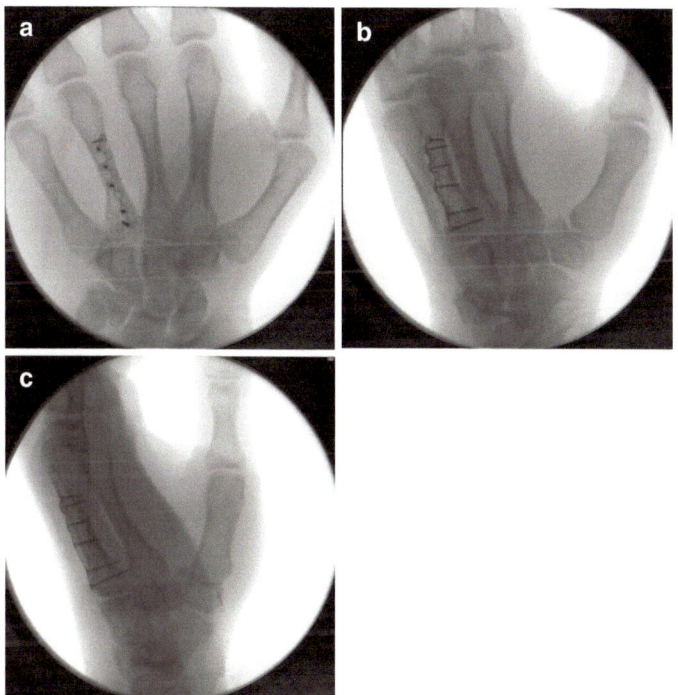

FIGURE 12.8 (**a–c**) Intraoperative final fluoroscopy PA and lateral views of a closed, left, spiral oblique fracture of the ring metacarpal status post open reduction internal fixation with a 1.5 mm low profile T-plate

Indications

Because of the presence of multiple oblique fractures and their inherent instability, operative treatment was pursued. Options include open or closed reduction and percutaneous pinning, open reduction with lag screw fixation, open reduction with plate fixation, and combined lag screw/plate fixation. For most metacarpal fractures reducible by closed means, CRPP is preferred. However, the presence of multiple fractures makes cross-pinning difficult. Antegrade or retro-

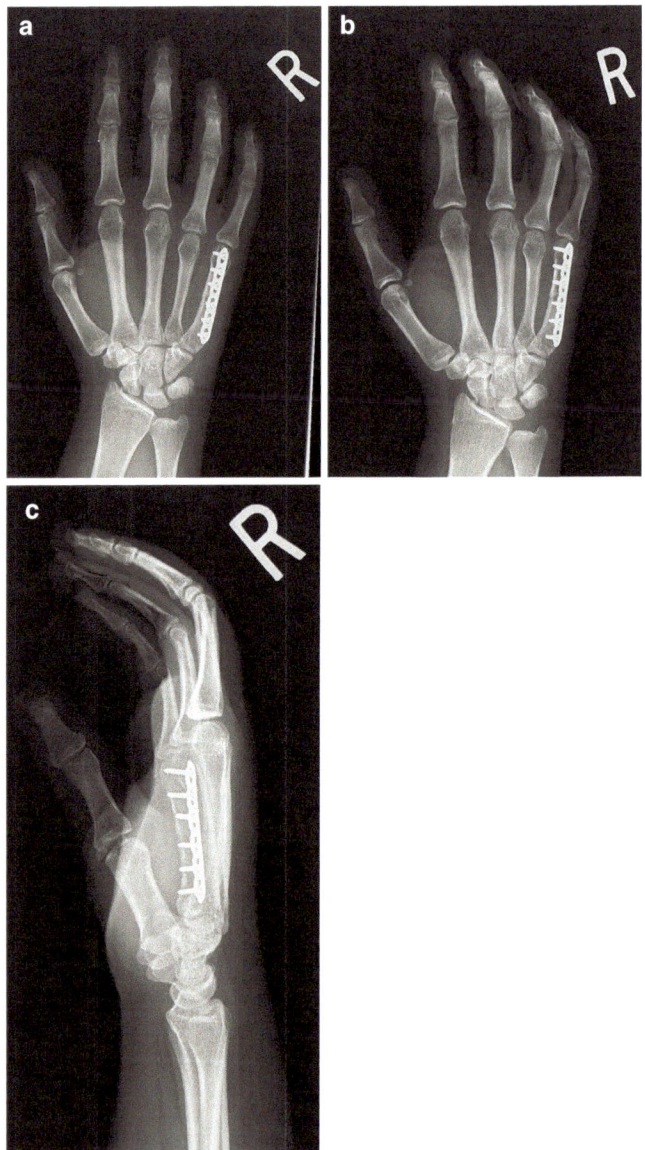

FIGURE 12.9 Three x-ray views of a right, transverse, small finger metacarpal fracture status post open reduction internal fixation with a conventional plate

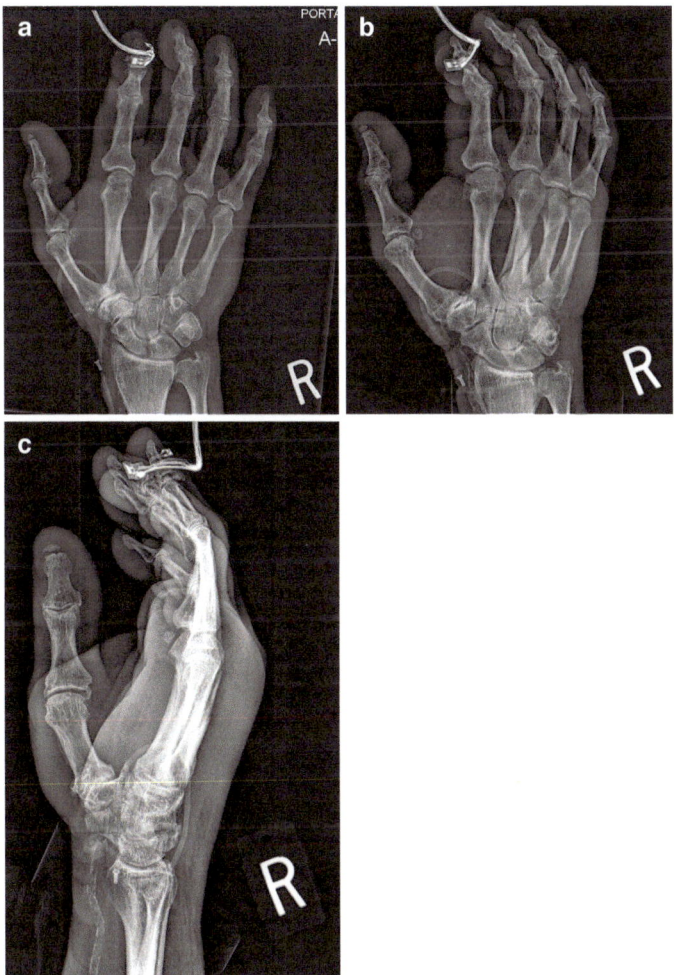

FIGURE 12.10 Three x-ray views of closed, long oblique, spiral fractures of the ring index, long and ring metacarpals

grade IM pinning remains an option. A decision was made to proceed with open fixation to allow for early mobilization without prominent hardware.

Description of Operation

Attention was first turned to the index finger metacarpal where traction and de-rotation reduced the fracture and a K-wire from the adjacent metacarpal held the reduction. An incision directly over the metacarpal allowed the placement of three 2.0 mm lag screws perpendicular to the fracture line (Fig. 12.11).

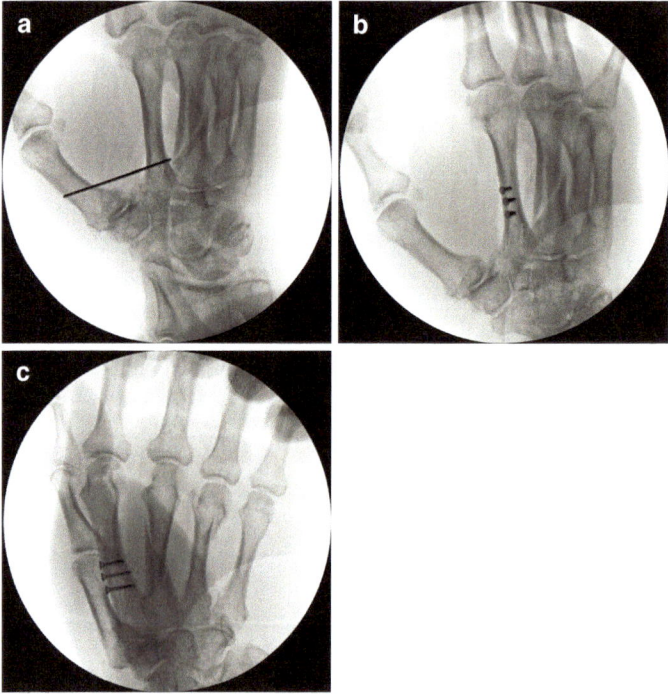

FIGURE 12.11 Intraoperative fluoroscopy oblique and PA views of a right index finger status post provisional reduction and pinning and subsequent placement of three 2.0 mm lag screws

An incision was made between the ring and long finger metacarpals. A large intercalary segment within the spiral fracture of the long finger was reduced with a 2.0 mm lag screw. A 1.5 mm low profile T-plate was then utilized to span the fracture. Images were obtained confirming fracture reduction, hardware placement, and lack of hardware prominence (Fig. 12.12).

The distal location of the ring finger fracture precluded plate fixation. The fracture was provisionally held with a K-wire placed percutaneously through the small finger metacarpal. Two 2.0 mm lag screws were placed across the fracture site (Fig. 12.12). The provisional K-wire was maintained for 2 weeks.

Post-operative Course

The patient was placed in an intrinsic plus volar splint. At 2 weeks post-op a custom wrist-based splint was fabricated. At 2 weeks post-op the ring finger pin was pulled.

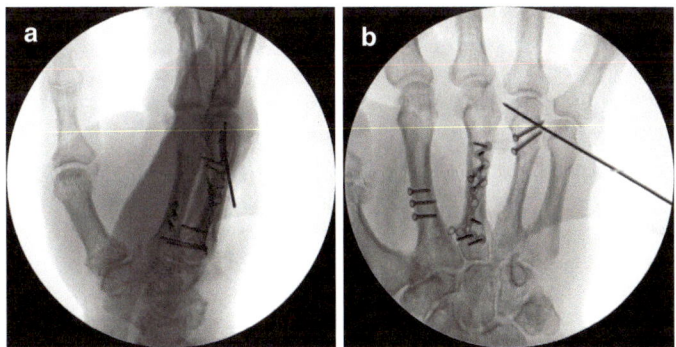

FIGURE 12.12 Intraoperative final fluoroscopy PA and lateral views of closed right index finger metacarpal fracture status post open reduction internal fixation with 2.0 mm lag screws, long finger metacarpal fracture status post open reduction internal fixation with a low profile 1.5 mm T-plate, and open reduction internal fixation of distal ring finger metacarpal fracture with 2.0 mm lag screws and a provisional K-wire

Case 5: Retrograde Headless Compression Screw Fixation

History

A 58-year-old right-hand-dominant female status post motor vehicle crash presented with left long, ring, and small metacarpal neck fractures (Fig. 12.13).

Indications

The patient was initially placed into a volar splint with further angulation noted at 2 weeks follow-up (Fig. 12.14). A decision was made to proceed with operative management. Treatment options include closed reduction percutaneous pinning, open reduction with retrograde headless compression screws, open reduction with plate fixation, or open reduction with a cerclage wire technique.

Description of Operation

A longitudinal incision was made between the long and ring metacarpals distally and the ring finger fracture exposed. The fragment was reduced using a pointed reduction clamp. A guidewire for a 3.0 mm headless compression screw was placed retrograde through the metacarpal head into the IM canal. The screw length was measured, the guidewire over-drilled, and the screw placed with the screw recessed 2 mm below the articular surface (Fig. 12.15).

The long finger metacarpal fracture was noted to be significantly comminuted precluding the use of a retrograde headless compression screw. A large radial-sided intraarticular fragment was secured with a 1.5 mm lag screw followed by placement of two 26-gauge wires as cerclage fixation. An incision slightly ulnar to the small finger metacarpal was made, the fracture visualized and reduced. Due to concerns

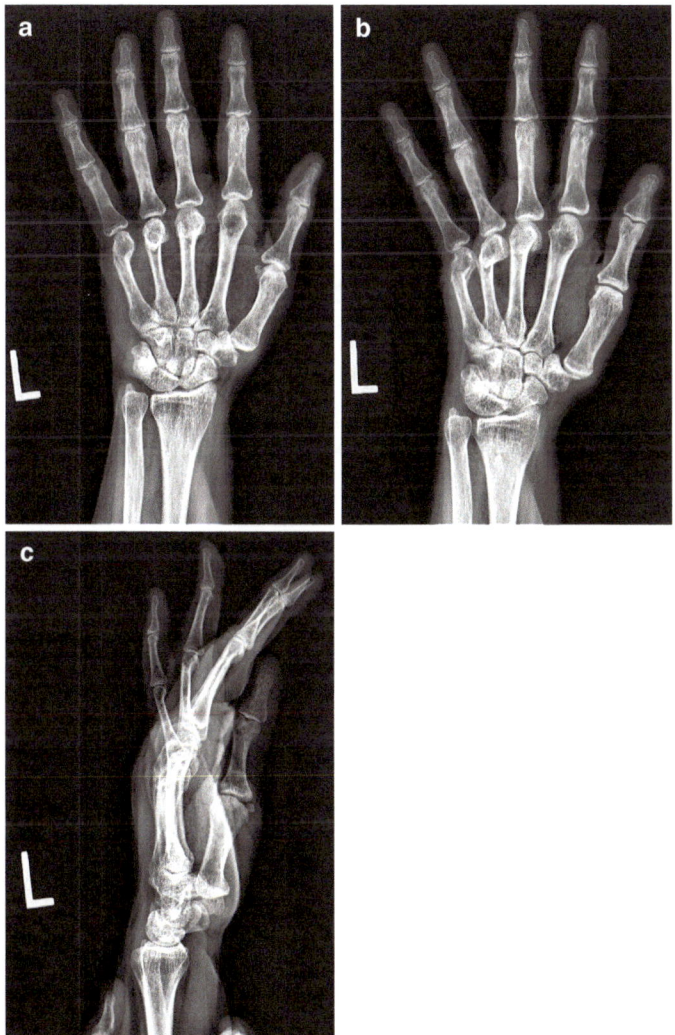

FIGURE 12.13 Three x-ray views of closed left long, ring, and small metacarpal neck fractures

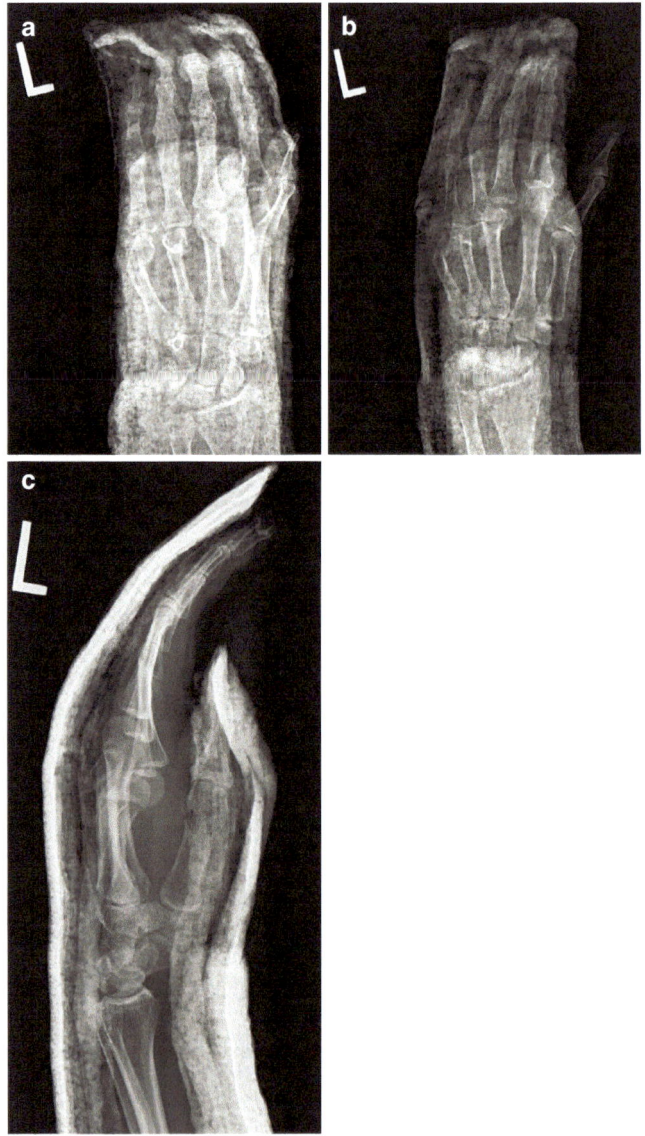

FIGURE 12.14 Three x-ray views of closed left long, ring, and small metacarpal neck fractures 2 weeks status post splinting with further angulation

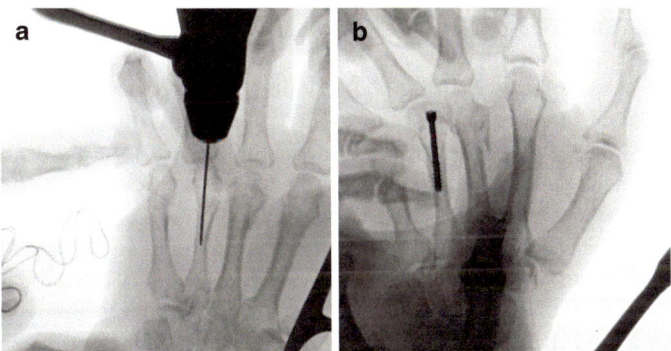

FIGURE 12.15 Intraoperative fluoroscopy PA and oblique views of a left ring finger metacarpal neck fracture status post placement of a guidewire for a 3.0 mm headless compression screw and subsequent placement of the screw

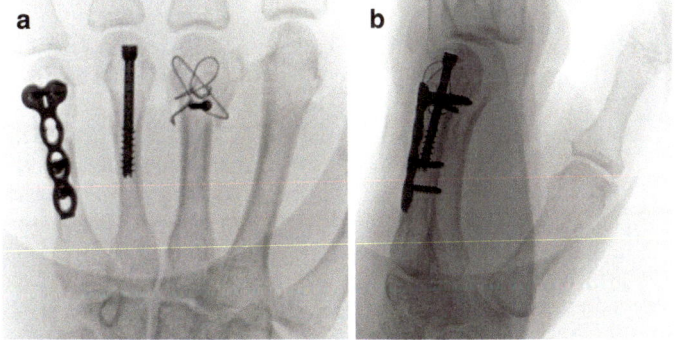

FIGURE 12.16 Intraoperative final fluoroscopy PA (**a**) and lateral (**b**) views of closed left long, ring, and small finger metacarpal neck fractures status post open reduction internal fixation with 1.5-mm lag screw fixation with supplementary cerclage wires for the middle finger, retrograde 3.0-mm headless compression screw for the ring finger, and a 2.0 mm locking plate for the small finger metacarpal neck fracture

with the narrow diameter of the small finger IM canal, a 2.0 mm locking plate was utilized to bridge the fracture (Fig. 12.16).

Post-operative Course

A volar splint was applied. At 10 days post-op the patient was placed into a custom splint and active motion initiated.

Metacarpal fractures are among the most common musculoskeletal injuries. Unstable metacarpal fractures can be challenging to treat. There is no specific technique that is superior, and there are many different techniques that are successful with each having its own advantages and disadvantages. Stable fixation that allows early motion remains the most important factor for preventing adhesions and improving outcomes. Ultimately it is important to consider the specific injury pattern in the context of individual patient factors to determine the appropriate treatment for each patient.

References

1. Chung KC, Spilson SV. The frequency and epidemiology of hand and forearm fractures in the United States. J Hand Surg Am. 2001;26:908–15.
2. Van Onselen EBH, Karim RB, Hage JJ, Ritt MJPF. Prevalence and distribution of hand fractures. J Hand Surg Br. 2003;28:491–5.
3. Taylor N, Chung KC. Extra-articular phalangeal and metacarpal fractures. In: Chung KC, Murray PM, editors. Hand surgery update V. Illinois: American Society for Surgery of the Hand; 2011. p. 7–17.
4. Stahl S, Schwartz O. Complication of K-wire fixation of fractures and dislocations in the hand and wrist. Arch Orthop Trauma Surg. 2001;212:527–30.

Chapter 13
Phalanx Fractures: Tips and Tricks

Kirsten A. Sumner and Joel Christian Klena

The operative and non-operative treatment of phalangeal fractures can be challenging. While fracture non-union is uncommon, adhesions and stiffness are common complications. There are three key principles to treating hand fractures: reduction within acceptable parameters, stable maintenance of reduction, and early mobilization [1]. While brief immobilization post-operatively is common practice, more than 3 weeks of immobilization leads to stiffness. We present several illustrative cases to demonstrate common strategies and pitfalls to avoid when treating these fractures.

K. A. Sumner (✉)
Department of Orthopaedic Surgery, Geisinger Medical Center, Danville, PA, USA
e-mail: kasumner@geisinger.edu

J. C. Klena
Division of Hand Surgery, Department of Orthopaedic Surgery, Geisinger Medical Center, Danville, PA, USA

© Springer Nature Switzerland AG 2020   199
D. S. Horwitz et al. (eds.), *Tips and Tricks for Problem Fractures, Volume I*,
https://doi.org/10.1007/978-3-030-38274-2_13

Case 1

History

A 56-year-old left-hand-dominant male struck his right hand against a wall and presented with a closed fracture of the small finger. A rotational deformity was present. X-rays (Fig. 13.1) revealed a right small finger spiral oblique fracture of the proximal phalanx (P1).

Indications

Maintaining reduction of spiral oblique fractures via closed means is difficult. Because of the rotational deformity a decision to proceed with operative treatment was made. Options for fixation include closed reduction and percutaneous pinning (CRPP), open reduction and pinning, open reduction and lag screw fixation, and open reduction with plate fixation. For most phalanx fractures, CRPP remains the preferred method of fixation. Advantages include minimizing scar formation and the ease of hardware removal. Should open reduction be necessary, either pin fixation or lag screw fixation are viable options. Because of the close association of the extensor tendon with the underlying phalanx, plate and screw fixation carries with it a high risk of hardware irritation, adhesions, and stiffness.

Description of Operation

The patient received LMA general anesthesia and was positioned supine with a hand table. A non-sterile tourniquet in the axilla was utilized. Initial radiographs were taken with longitudinal traction and counter-rotation applied to the digit. Care was taken to restore length and remove any rotational deformity. A lateral view of the digit demonstrating no rotation at *both* the PIP and DIP joints ensures restoration of normal rota-

FIGURE 13.1 Small
finger spiral oblique
fracture of the
proximal phalanx

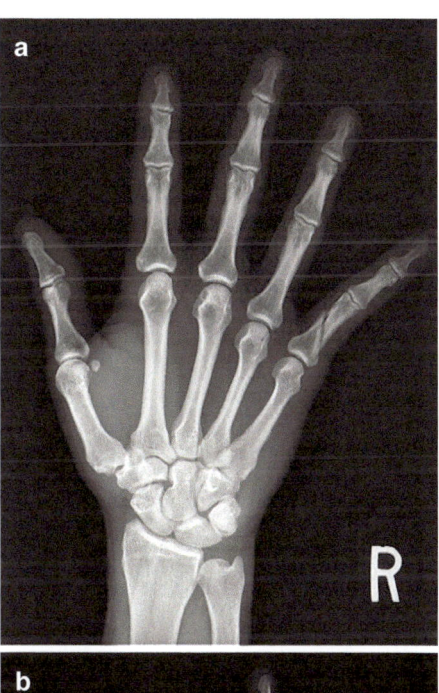

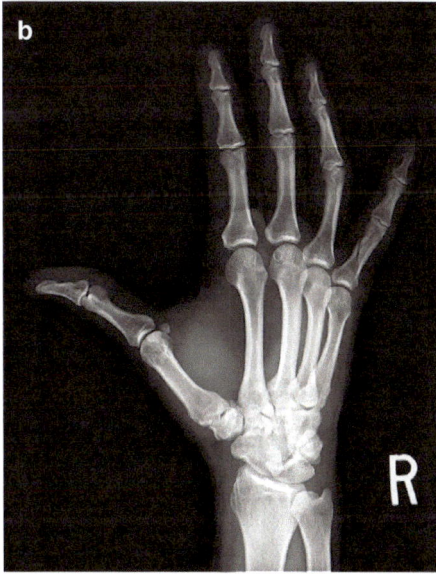

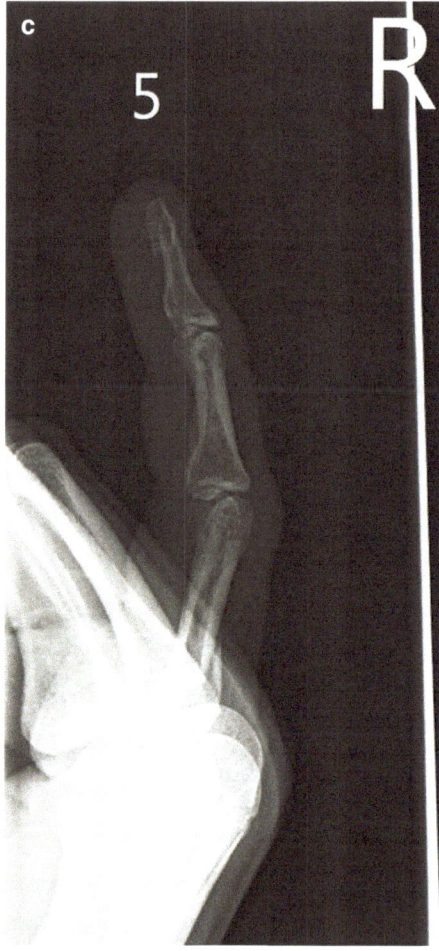

FIGURE 13.1 (continued)

tion at the fracture site (Fig. 13.2). Reduction was maintained with a percutaneous clamp followed by placement of two 0.045″ Kirschner wires (k-wires) perpendicular to the oblique fracture line. Pin placement was verified under multi-planar imaging (Fig. 13.3). An additional k-wire (0.035″) was placed to increase fracture stability and allow early motion (Fig. 13.4).

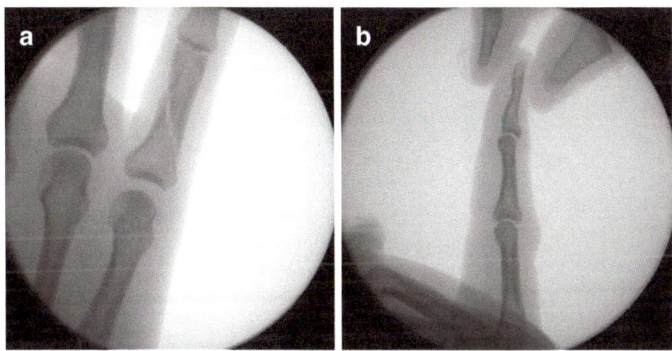

FIGURE 13.2 Longitudinal traction and counter-rotation applied to the digit demonstrated no rotational deformity

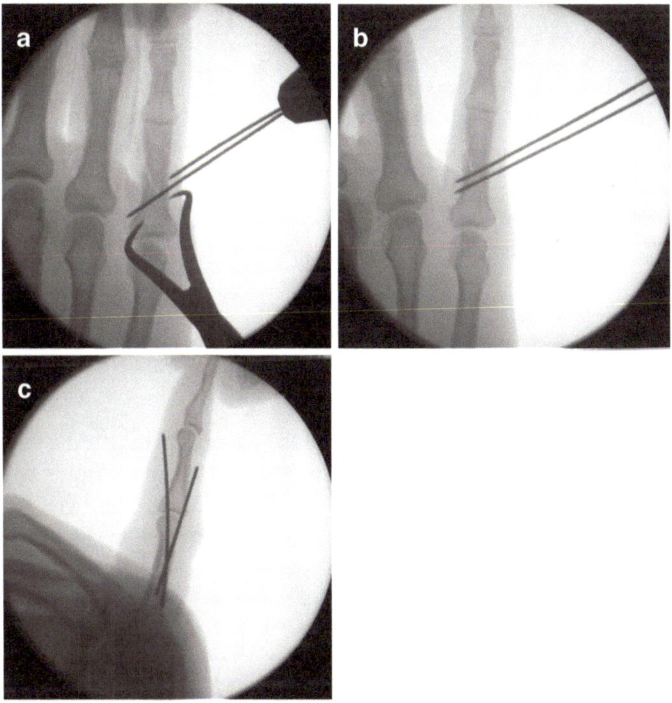

FIGURE 13.3 Two 0.045″ k-wires were placed perpendicular to the oblique fracture line

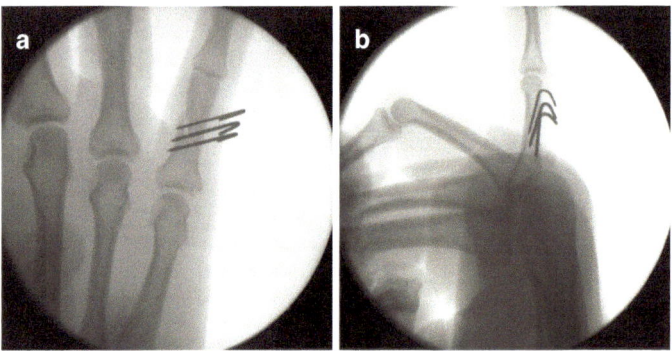

FIGURE 13.4 A third K-wire (0.035") was placed to increase fracture stability

Post-operative Course

The patient was placed in an ulnar gutter splint in the intrinsic plus position. He returned at day 5 post-operatively for a pin site check, fabrication of a hand-based custom splint for protection, and initiation of early motion. The pins remained in place for 4 weeks prior to being pulled in the office.

Case 2

History

A 43-year-old right-hand-dominant female presented with a transverse proximal phalanx fracture of the small finger with angulation on both the AP and lateral views. Characteristic apex volar angulation was seen on the lateral view (Fig. 13.5).

Indications

Treatment options include CRPP, ORIF with pin fixation, and ORIF with plate and screw fixation. Fractures at the base

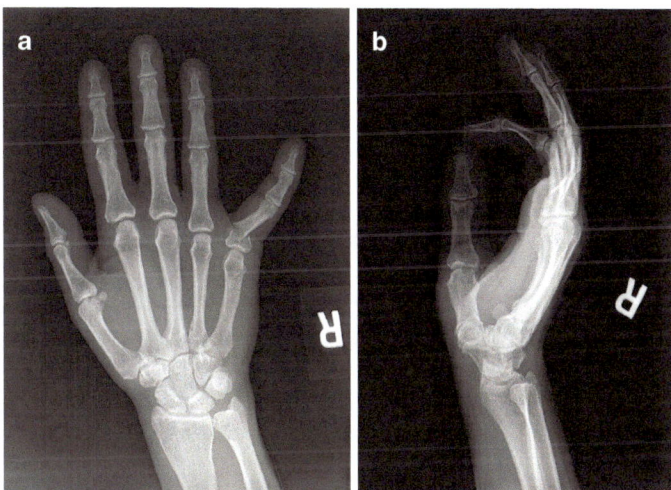

FIGURE 13.5 Transverse proximal phalanx fracture of the small finger with apex volar angulation

of P1 are particularly unforgiving with respect to scar formation and tendon adhesions; open fixation should be avoided. A decision was made to proceed with CRPP.

Description of Operation

Border digits are more amenable to CRPP than their central counterparts. A key to reducing P1 base fractures involves correcting the apex volar angular deformity by placing the digit in the intrinsic plus position (MCP flexion and PIP extension). Two 0.045″ k-wires were placed antegrade in a cross-pinning fashion (Fig. 13.6).

Post-operative Course

The patient was placed in an ulnar gutter splint in the intrinsic plus position. She returned on post-operative day 5 for pin

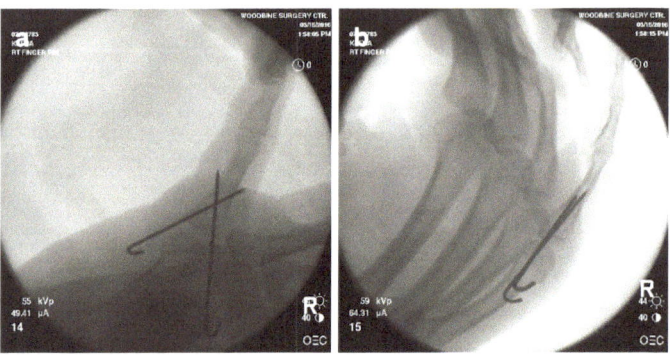

FIGURE 13.6 Two 0.045″ k-wires were placed antegrade in a cross-pinning fashion

site check, a custom splint, and initiation of gentle motion. Motion was advanced as tolerated at week 2 post-op. The pins were removed at 4 weeks.

Case 3

History

A 72-year-old right-hand-dominant female was involved in a motor vehicle collision with x-rays demonstrating a small finger transverse proximal phalanx fracture with characteristic apex volar angulation (Fig. 13.7). The patient was placed in a poorly molded ulnar gutter splint with the MP and PIP joints in extension. Severe concomitant injuries delayed the patient's presentation for definitive management until 2 weeks post-injury. X-rays obtained at that time revealed further displacement and angulation of the fracture (Fig. 13.8).

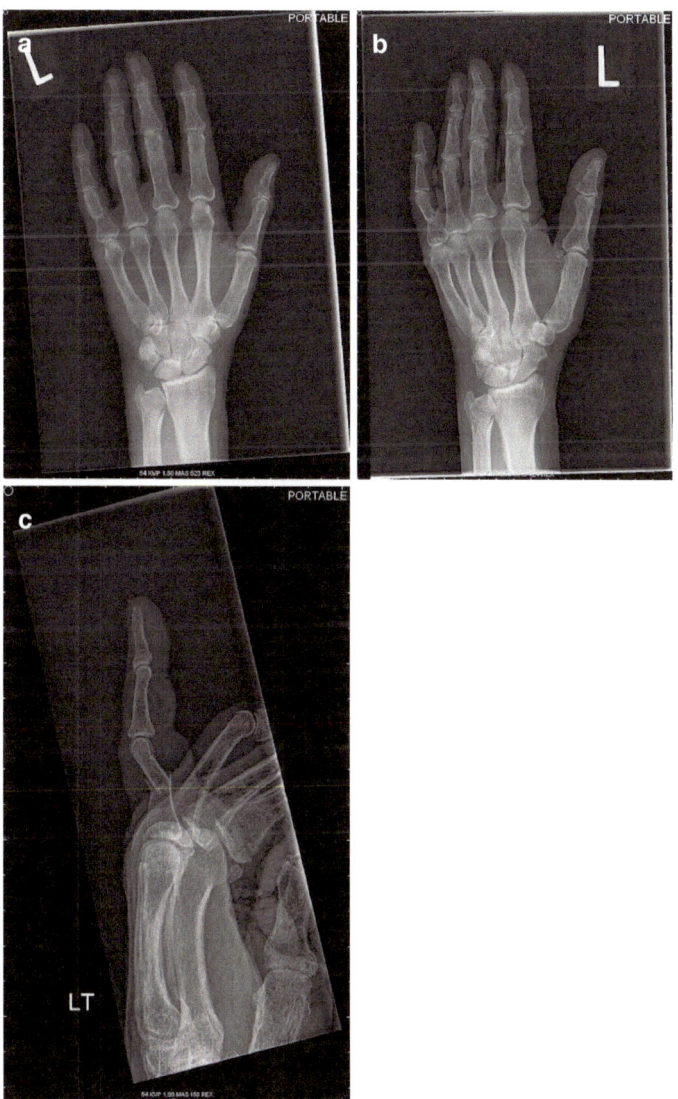

FIGURE 13.7 Small finger transverse proximal phalanx fracture with characteristic apex volar angulation

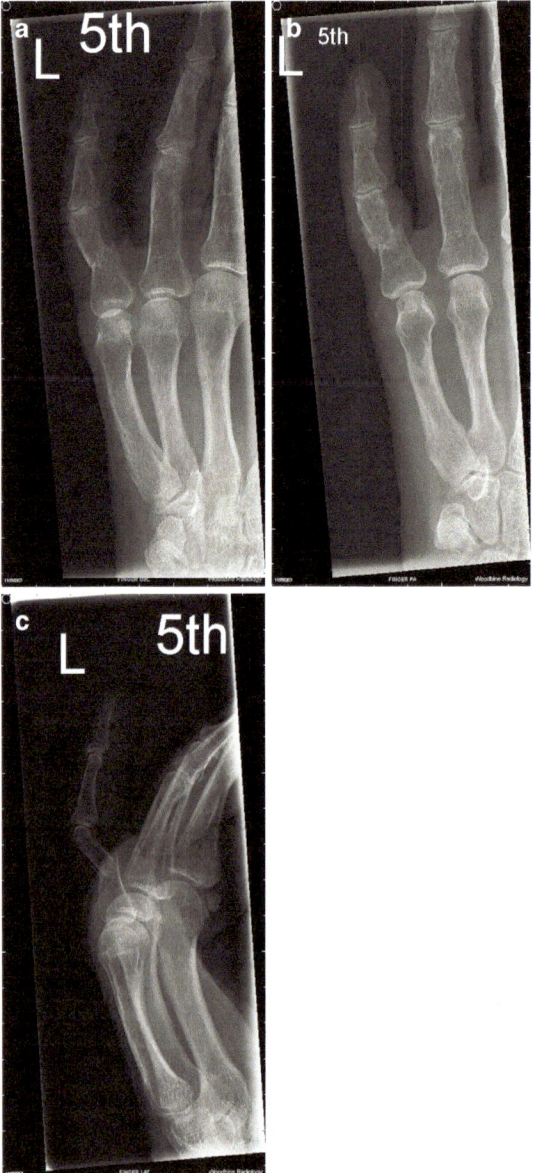

FIGURE 13.8 Further displacement and angulation of the fracture 2 weeks post-injury

Indications

Delayed presentation of a displaced and angulated small finger proximal phalanx fracture can be a contraindication for surgery. Prolonged immobilization pre-operatively places the patient at a significant risk for stiffness following surgery. This patient would have benefited from initial treatment in a splint molded to place the digit in the intrinsic plus position to reduce the apex volar deformity. Splinting the digit loosely distally to the adjacent ring finger would help reduce both angulation and translation on the AP view.

Description of Operation

The patient underwent initial attempts at CRPP. Under multi-planar imaging, the digit was placed in the intrinsic plus position and longitudinal traction applied. Significant comminution prevented an anatomic reduction from being achieved. A decision was made to proceed with open fixation. A curvilinear dorsal incision was made over the fracture site with care taken to identify and protect the extensor tendon. The large comminuted segment made spanning bridge plate fixation the best fixation option. A low-profile, 1.5 mm 6-hole stacked plate was chosen. The plate was affixed distally with the position of the plate offset slightly ulnar on the dorsum of the phalanx to minimize contact with the overlying extensor tendon. Longitudinal traction was applied to the digit with the MP joint flexed, length and rotation were verified under multi-planar imaging, and the plate was fixed proximally (Fig. 13.9). Proximally, the transverse fibers and lateral band from the intrinsic contribution to the extensor tendon overlie the plate and are a potential source of tendon adhesions. Resection of the proximal portion of the intrinsic tendons is necessary.

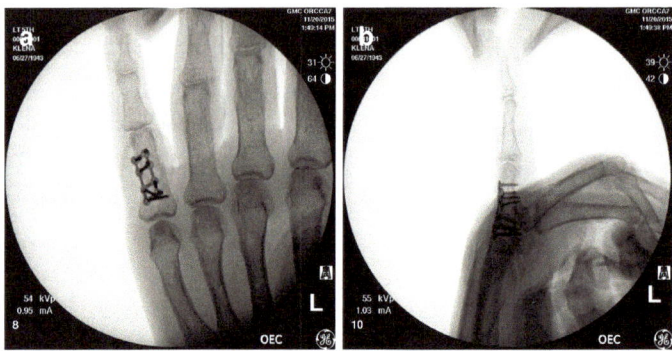

FIGURE 13.9 Dorsal plate fixation was performed due to inability to close reduce the fracture with the amount of comminution present

Post-operative Course

The patient was placed in an ulnar gutter splint in the intrinsic plus position. She returned on post-op day 5 for a custom hand-based splint and initiation of motion. Despite aggressive early motion, the patient underwent a subsequent tenolysis and hardware removal for stiffness and ultimately achieved only a modest outcome.

Case 4

History

A 15-year-old right-hand-dominant female sustained a closed, bicondylar intra-articular fracture of the middle phalanx (P2) of the ring finger playing flag football (Fig. 13.10).

Indications

Unicondylar and bicondylar phalangeal fractures are unstable and require operative intervention. An argument can be

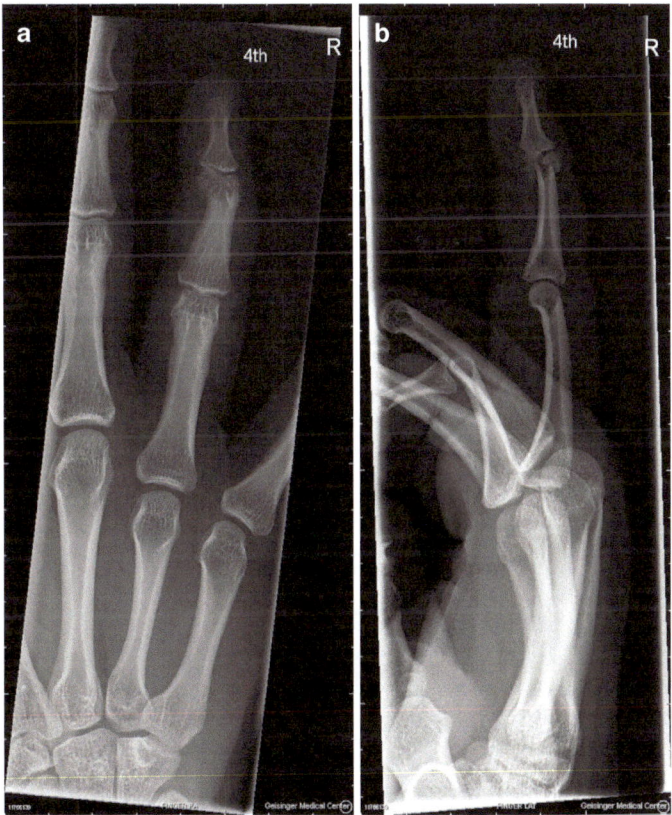

FIGURE 13.10 Bicondylar fracture of the middle phalanx of the ring finger

made to operatively treat even non-displaced fractures due to their inherent instability [2]. These fractures are typically amenable to CRPP.

Description of Operation

Under multi-planar imaging, closed reduction of the fracture was achieved. Longitudinal traction can be applied manually or with a pointed reduction clamp applied to the distal phalanx. A second clamp is applied at the fracture site and alignment verified on both AP and lateral views (Fig. 13.11). Fixation of the fracture was achieved with two 0.045″ k-wires. The initial wire is placed transversely across the two condyles converting the three-part fracture into a two-part fracture. A second k-wire is then placed obliquely to reduce the bicondylar fragment to the proximal portion of the phalanx (Fig. 13.12).

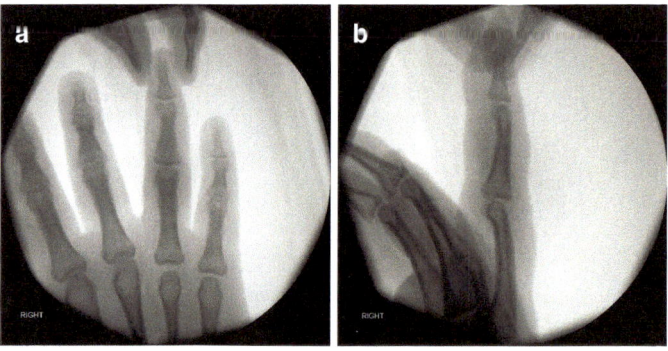

FIGURE 13.11 Closed reduction of the fracture was achieved

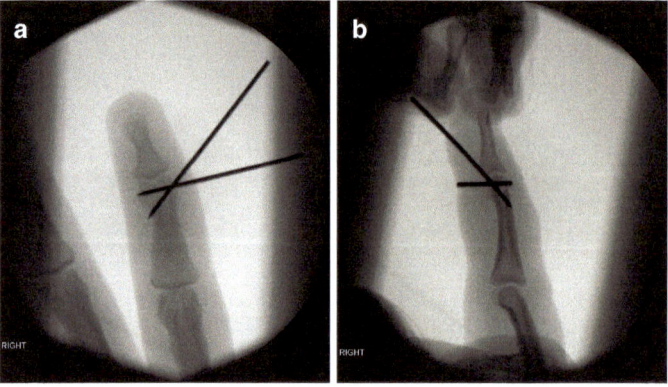

FIGURE 13.12 Two 0.045″ k-wire fixation: initial wire transverse across the condyles followed by a second oblique k-wire

Post-operative Course

A volar splint in the intrinsic plus position was placed in the operating room. The patient returned post-op day 7 for a pin site check, fabrication of a hand-based custom splint, and initiation of gentle motion at the MCP and PIP joints. Motion at the DIP joint was initiated following pin removal at 3 weeks post-op.

Case 5

History

A 24-year-old right-hand-dominant male injured his left index finger playing basketball and presented with a closed, comminuted intra-articular fracture of the volar base of the middle phalanx (Fig. 13.13).

Indications

Impaction injuries of the PIP joint are often referred to as pilon fractures. They vary in severity depending on the force of injury and the degree of flexion at the PIP joint at the time of injury. Goals of treatment include restoring stability for early motion and maintaining articular congruency. As seen with this patient, the articular surface is often comminuted and not amenable to direct fixation techniques. An alternative treatment is dynamic traction via percutaneous pins. Several pin configurations are available including those using rubber bands for adjustable tension. We prefer the use of simple pins as described by Gaul and Rosenberg then modified by Badia et al. [3, 4].

Description of Operation

Under direct multiplanar imaging, longitudinal traction was applied. A dorsally directed force applied at the base of the middle phalanx provided further reduction of the articular

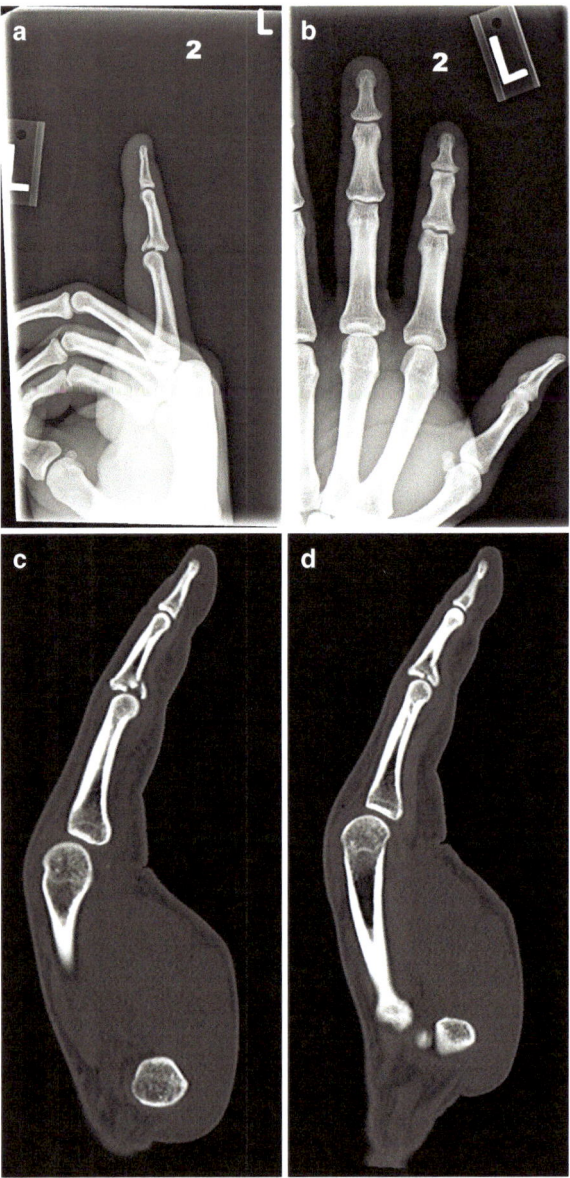

FIGURE 13.13 Comminuted intra-articular fracture of the volar base of the middle phalanx of the index finger

fragments. Alternatively, a percutaneous k-wire can be used as a joystick to provide direct reduction. A lateral view of the digit allows placement of a transverse 0.045″ k-wire through the center of rotation of both the proximal phalanx and the distal phalanx heads. The k-wires are bent 1 cm from the skin at a 90-degree angle. A second retrograde bend is placed in the proximal wire 1 cm beyond its intersection point with the distal wire providing a "seat" for the distal wire under traction (Fig. 13.14). The traction can be adjusted by adjusting the proximal/distal position of the "seat" formed for the distal transverse wire. Additional transverse pins can be incorporated in the middle phalanx to provide volar or dorsal translational forces at the PIP joint. A free arc of motion with concentric PIP joint motion was visualized radiographically from full extension to 90 degrees of flexion. A well-padded volar splint was applied.

Post-operative Course

The patient returned on post-operative day 3 for a hand-based, custom splint and initiation of range of motion exercises. The pins are removed in the clinic at post-operative week 4.

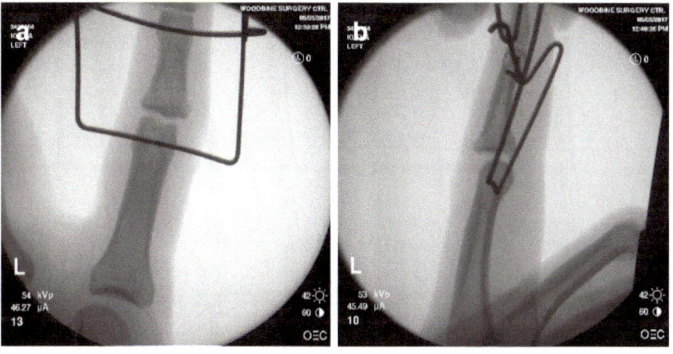

FIGURE 13.14 Dynamic traction with percutaneous pins

Phalanx fractures remain challenging to treat with high rates of stiffness. While the mainstay of treatment remains CRPP, surgeons must be aware of alternative techniques with the goal of achieving sufficient stability to allow early digital motion.

References

1. Taylor N, Chung KC. Extra-articular phalangeal and metacarpal fractures. In: Chung KC, Murray PM, editors. Hand surgery update V. Illinois: American Society for Surgery of the Hand; 2011. p. 7–17.
2. Weiss AP, Hastings H 2nd. Distal unicondylar fractures of the proximal phalanx. J Hand Surg Am. 1993;18:594–9.
3. Gaul JS Jr, Rosenberg SN. Fracture-dislocation of the middle phalanx at the proximal interphalangeal joint: repair with a simple intradigital traction-fixation device. Am J Orthop. 1998;27(10):682–8.
4. Badia A, Riano F, Ravikoff J, et al. Dynamic intradigital external fixation for proximal interphalangeal joint fracture dislocations. J Hand Surg Am. 2005;30(1):154–60.

Index

© Springer Nature Switzerland AG 2020   217
D. S. Horwitz et al. (eds.), *Tips and Tricks for Problem
Fractures, Volume I*,
https://doi.org/10.1007/978-3-030-38274-2